MANAGEMENT OF HYPERTENSION

by

Norman M. Kaplan, M.D.

Department of Internal Medicine
University of Texas
Southwestern Medical School
5323 Harry Hines Boulevard
Dallas, Texas 75235

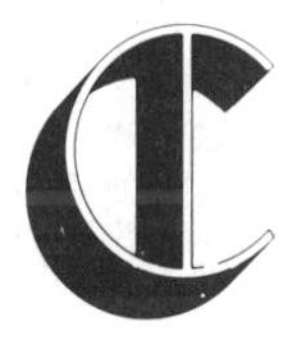

AVAILABLE FROM:
CREATIVE INFOMATICS, INC.
P.O. BOX 1607
DURANT, OK 74702-1607

CREATIVE INFOMATICS, INC.
P.O. BOX 1607
DURANT, OK 74702-1607
(405) 924-0643

First Edition Published in the United States 1986
Published Simultaneously in Canada

ISBN: 0-917634-22-5

Printed in the United States of America
Library of Congress Catalog Card Number:
86-070813

Table of Contents

Tables

Figures

Foreword

This book, hopefully, will prove useful to those who want a ready up-to-date reference to practical issues in the treatment of hypertensive patients. My larger book, Clinical Hypertension, now in its 4th edition, should provide additional background, detail, and references for those who need them.

I thank all of my co-workers, both in Dallas and elsewhere, who have provided me with the data and the insights needed to write this book.

#1 Measurement of Blood Pressure

The first and most important step in the management of hypertension is a careful assessment of the level of the blood pressure. It must be taken frequently and carefully. The blood pressure naturally varies a great deal so it is important to avoid all controllable causes of variation. During 24 hour ambulatory monitoring, pressures while awake may vary by more than 30 mm Hg, with highest levels usually noted in the early morning and lower readings in the afternoon. Much lower levels are usual during sleep, with the important exception of higher readings during periods of sleep apnea.

GENERAL PRINCIPLES

To Establish the Diagnosis

At least 3 sets of 3 readings should be taken with intervals of 2 weeks or more between each set unless the initial level is so high (above 200/120) or target organ damage is so ominous as to demand immediate intervention. Even more readings may be fruitfully obtained from self-taken home measurements, preferably at various times and under various circumstances.

Levels of blood pressure tend to fall after the first reading with most of the fall noted during the first few weeks. Most home readings are 5-10 mm Hg lower than those obtained in the office.

Even though the initial higher office readings may indicate higher risks for the subsequent development of cardiovascular disease, the average of multiple readings taken over 1 to 2 months should be taken to establish the diagnosis of hypertension and to decide upon the need for therapy.

To Monitor Progress

For most, only occassional followup readings are needed, initially more frequently than later. If changes in therapy are made, readings should be taken after 2 to 4 weeks, unless side effects occur. Once the goal of therapy is reached and the patient is asymptomatic, readings need only be obtained every 4 to 6 months.

Those whose pressures remain above 140/90 mm Hg should be monitored more frequently as their therapy is altered. Some who seem to respond poorly on the basis of office readings may be found to be well controlled by home readings.

Basic Technique

The basic technique in the measurement of the blood pressure includes:

- Three readings at each visit
- On initial visit supine and standing readings may be indicated
- Measure blood pressure in both arms; if there is a persistent difference, use arm with higher pressure
- The patient should sit in a chair for at least 5 minutes with the arm unconstricted and supported at the level of the heart on a platform or table
- Avoid (or if unavoidable, make note of) extraneous factors which may alter pressure
  - Smoking or eating within the prior 30 minutes
  - Anxiety

- Talking
- Exertion
- Cold
- Medications, which include:
  - Estrogens
  - Adrenal steroids
  - Adrenergic drugs such as nose drops or 10% phenylephrine used to dilate pupils for funduscopic exam
- Bladder distension

- Note the time of day
- Use proper sized cuff: the largest that will fit the upper arm is appropriate
- Inflate bladder to above systolic level by palpating the disappearance of the radial pulse. If radial artery remains palpable after pulse disappears, consider "pseudohypertension" from calcified vessels which cannot be collapsed beneath bladder
- Deflate cuff at rate of 2-3 mm Hg per heart beat
- Use disappearance of sound (Korotkoff V) as diastolic level
- In patients below age 20 or if femoral pulse is weak, take pressure in one leg

(from Kaplan, NM: Clinical Hypertension, 4th ed, 1986).

References:

Cottier C, Julius S, Gajendragadkar SV, Schork A: Usefulness of home BP determination in treating borderline hypertension. JAMA 1982;248:555-8.

Mancia G, Bertinieri G, Grassi G, et al.: Effects of blood-pressure measurements by the doctor on patient's blood pressure and heart rate. Lancet 1983;2:695-8.

O'Brien E, Fitzgerald D, O'Malley K: Blood pressure measurement: current practice and future trends. Br Med J 1985;290:729-34.

Perloff D, Sokolow M, Cowan R: The prognostic value of ambulatory blood pressure. JAMA 1983;249:2792-8.

#2 Definition of Hypertension

The long-term risks for the development of cardiovascular disease increase with every increment of blood pressure. The degree of risk for coronary and cerebral vascular disease is some 2-fold higher in adults with diastolic blood pressure (DBP) above 90 mm Hg compared to those with DBP below 80. The definition of hypertension is usually based on DBP but the presence of isclated elevations of systolic blood pressure (SBP) above 160 mm Hg, usually seen in people over age 65, is associated with a significantly higher risk, particularly for stroke.

Based on the relative increase in risks, hypertension may be defined as sustained average levels of blood pressure above 140/90 mm Hg in adult patients. Those with DBP below 90 but SBP above 160 may be defined as having isolated systolic hypertension. These levels have been proposed as the upper limit of normal for children:

Age	Blood Pressure
14-18	135/90
10-14	125/85
6-10	120/80
Below 6	110/75

Classification by Degree

The 1984 Joint National Committee report proposed this classification of the degree of hypertension:

Range of Blood Pressure	Category of Hypertension
Diastolic	
90-104	Mild hypertension
105-114	Moderate hypertension
115 and above	Severe hypertension
Systolic (DBP < 90)	
140-159	Borderline isolated systolic hypertension
160 and above	Isolated systolic hypertension

The relative frequency of various categories of diastolic hypertension in a large population of people screened at home by the Hypertension Detection and Followup Program was about 80% mild, 15% moderate and 5% severe (Figure 1).

Those patients with DBP from 85 to 89 mm Hg may be classified as "high-normal." They should be more frequently re-checked and counseled more vigorously to follow the non-drug modalities (see Sections 9 and 10) which may decrease the likelihood for the progression of hypertension. Even if they do not, they should improve overall cardiovascular status at no financial cost and little interference with current life style. Cessation of smoking, although it will not lower blood pressure, is the single most beneficial move to improve cardiovascular health.

An Operational Definition

More than the risks of various levels of blood pressure should be considered before labeling a person as hypertensive. Logically, the label should be affixed only if active therapy is indicated.

People labeled as hypertensive may suffer from increased psychoneurotic and other complaints, resulting in an increase in absenteeism from work. In addition, the label may be responsible for added economic burdens, e.g. higher life insurance premiums and loss of job opportunities.

There is, then, a need to balance the risks of not diagnosing and treating a level of blood pressure against the costs and risks of doing so. In addition to the costs of labeling, there are risks from all currently used antihypertensive drugs. On the basis of current knowledge, most authorities agree that drug therapy be given to those with average DBP above 95 mm Hg, although some advocate that the level should be as low as 90 and by others as high as 100 or even 105 (see Section 11).

From an operational viewpoint, many who are at increased risk need not be diagnosed as "hypertensive." However, they should be more carefully monitored and more vigorously counseled to improve their unhealthy life style. The label should be affixed to all with DBP that remains above 95 and, logically, to elderly with SBP above 160. Those with DBP between 85 and 94 or SBP between 140 and 159 who have few other risk factors may be more appropriately called "borderline" or "high-normal."

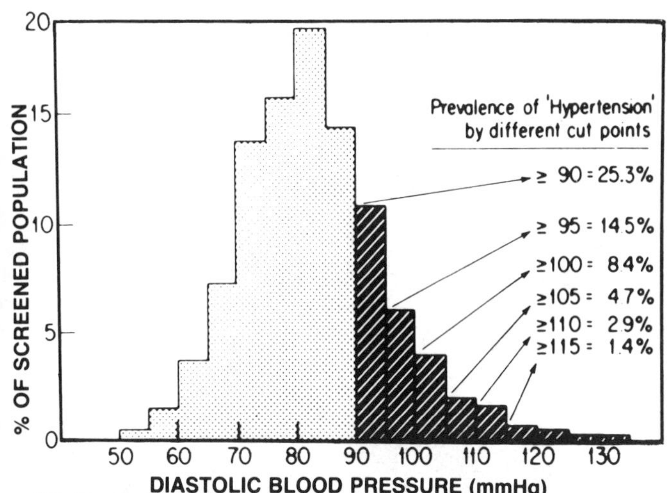

FIGURE 1. Frequency distribution of diastolic blood pressure at home screen (158,906 persons; 30 to 69 years of age). (From The Hypertension Detection and Follow-up Program. Circulation Research 40 (Supp I):106,1977, by permission of the American Heart Association, Inc.)

References:

Joint National Committee on Detection, Evaluation, and Treatment of High Blood Pressure: The 1984 report of the Joint National Committee on Detection, Evaluation, and Treatment of High Blood Pressure. Arch Intern Med 1984;144:1045-57.

Lichtenstein MJ, Shipley MJ, Rose G: Systolic and diastolic blood pressures as predictors of coronary heart disease mortality in the Whitehall Study. Br Med J 1985;291:243-5.

MacDonald LA, Sackett DL, Haynes RB, Taylor DW: Labelling in hypertension: a review of the behavioural and psychological consequences. J Chron Dis 1984;37:933-42.

Subcommittee on Definition and Prevalence of the 1984 Joint National Committee: Hypertension prevalence and the status of awareness, treatment, and control in the United States. Hypertension 1985;7:457-68.

#3 Types of Hypertension

3.

Primary

In typical clinical practice, 95% of hypertensive adults aged 18 to 65 will have no identifiable cause, thus their hypertension should be defined either as primary or essential or idiopathic.

Secondary

The frequency of the secondary forms will likely approximate these figures:

- Renal parenchymal disease — 3 to 4%
- Renal vascular hypertension — 0.5 to 1%
- Adrenal hyperfunction — 0.1 to 0.3%
  - Pheochromocytoma
  - Cushing's syndrome
  - Primary aldosteronism
- Miscellaneous causes — 0.1 to 0.3%

Special Populations

Populations composed of varying proportions of special groups of patients will have different frequencies than those listed above.

Adults with Severe or Resistant Hypertension: Those with accelerated (Grade 3 fundi) or malignant (Grade 4 fundi) hypertension or whose hypertension remains resistant to appropriate therapy have a higher frequency of renal parenchymal disease and, even more so, of renal vascular hypertension. The frequency of renal vascular hypertension may be as high as 33% in such patients (see Section 5).

Women Taking Oral Contraceptives: After starting estrogen-containing oral contraceptives, most women experience a 2-4 mm Hg increase in blood pressure. As many as 5% of previously normotensive women will have a rise of DBP above 90 mm Hg after 5 years of pill use, a rate 2-3 times higher than women not taking the pill. Why the blood pressure rises more in some women is unknown but they may have a preexisting propensity to develop primary hypertension or underlying renal dysfunction (see Section 7).

Children: Pre-pubertal hypertensive children most likely have a renal cause. Post-pubertal children most likely have primary hypertension but a higher frequency of certain secondary causes is seen among them (see Section 30).

Elderly: Those who have the onset of hypertension after age 50 and even more so after age 60 have a higher frequency of renal parenchymal disease and renovascular hypertension.

References:

Danielson M, Dammstrom B-G: The prevalence of secondary and curable hypertension. Acta Med Scand 1981;209:451-5.

Lewin A, Blaufox MD, Castle H, Entwisle G, Langford H: Apparent prevalence of curable hypertension in the Hypertension Detection and Follow-up Program. Arch Intern Med 1985;145:424-7.

Rudnick KV, Sackett DL, Hirst S, Holmes C: Hypertension in a family practice. Can Med Assoc J 1977;117:492-7.

#4 Primary Hypertension

4.

Background

The specific cause is unknown. A genetic predisposition has been documented with about a 2-fold higher incidence in those with a close relative who is hypertensive. Environmental factors which increase the incidence include:

- obesity
- psychogenic stress
- high sodium intake

Various defects in the transport of sodium across cell membranes and a higher intracellular concentration of sodium and calcium may be involved.

The disease usually appears between ages 30 and 50, is slowly progressive and remains asymptomatic until significant target organ damage appears after 10 to 20 years.

Evaluation

For the majority of adult and adolescent hypertensive patients, the following evaluation should be done to assess target organ damage, to rule out secondary causes and to ascertain the overall cardiovascular risk status:

- Hematocrit
- Urine analysis
- Automated blood chemistry
  - creatinine
  - fasting glucose
  - sodium
  - potassium
  - total cholesterol
  - HDL-cholesterol
- Electrocardiogram

TABLE 1
OVERALL GUIDELINES FOR EVALUATION

Diagnosis	*Diagnostic Procedure* Initial	Additional
Chronic renal disease	Urinalysis, BUN or creatinine, sonography	Renin assay, renal biopsy, IVP
Renovascular disease	Bruit, plasma renin	Aortogram, renal vein renins
Coarctation	Blood pressure in legs	Aortogram
Primary aldosteronism	Plasma potassium	Urinary potassium, plasma renin, plasma or urinary aldosterone
Cushing's syndrome	A.M. plasma cortisol after 1 mg dexamethasone at bedtime	Urinary 17-OCHCS after variable doses of dexamethasone
Pheochromocytoma	Spot urine for metanephrine	Urinary VMA and catechols; plasma catechols, basal and after 0.3 mg clonidine

Additional tests may be needed for those in the previously noted special populations or who display suggestive features of a secondary cause by history or physical examination (Table 1).

In the near future, two additional procedures may be more frequently indicated, based upon current evidence, which shows that they are more sensitive indices of the severity of hypertension: echocardiography, which shows left ventricular hypertrophy much earlier than does electrocardiography and 24-hour ambulatory blood pressure monitoring, which has been found to predict more accurately the development of target organ damage than by the levels obtained by repeated office measurements.

References:

Devereux RB: Echocardiography: state of the art - 1984. Cardiol 1984;71:118-35.

Epstein AM, Hartley RM, Charlton JR, Harris CM, Jarman B, McNeil BJ: A comparison of ambulatory test ordering for hypertensive patients in the United States and England. JAMA 1984;252:1723-6.

Kwan CY: Dysfunction of calcium handling by smooth muscle in hypertension. Can J Physiol Pharmacol 1985;63:366-74.

Notes

#5 Secondary Hypertension: Renal

Renal parenchymal and vascular diseases are the most common causes of secondary hypertension, particularly in children, the elderly, and those with severe or resistant disease.

5.

RENAL PARENCHYMAL DISEASE

A considerable percentage of patients, as many as 10%, who start with primary hypertension develop progressive nephrosclerosis and end up with chronic renal failure. This course is more common among black hypertensives and those who have co-existing diabetes mellitus or poorly controlled hypertension.

As renal function deteriorates, hypertension becomes more prevalent and is present in about 85% of those with end-stage renal disease (ESRD). In such patients, it may not be possible to dissect cause from effect but renal function is normal in most with primary hypertension whose blood pressure is well controlled, whereas renal dysfunction (proteinuria, elevated serum creatinine, lower GFR) is prominent even without significant hypertension in most with a renal cause.

Clinical Features

The blood pressure tends to rise as renal function is lost, mainly from the inability of the damaged kidneys to excrete sodium and water. In some, renin hypersecretion is responsible and the absence of normal renal vasodepressor hormones may be involved.

All forms of progressive renal disease may lead to hypertension. Patients with polycystic disease may more frequently be hypertensive, those with analgesic nephropathy less frequently. Vasculitis, as seen with collagen vascular diseases, may induce acute, severe renal failure.

Pyelonephritis is rarely a factor except in patients with reflux nephropathy. Diabetic nephropathy is becoming more prevalent as more patients with diabetes live for 20 years or longer after developing the disease.

Management

The effective control of hypertension may slow and even partially reverse the progress of renal failure. Control may be accomplished by reduction in fluid volume by restriction of dietary sodium, high doses of loop diuretics or dialysis. More potent antihypertensive agents, in particular minoxidil, may be particularly useful (see Section 33). In experimental models, converting enzyme inhibitors provide special protection against progression of renal damage. In the future, atrial natriuretic factor (atriopeptin) may be of even greater benefit.

RENAL VASCULAR HYPERTENSION (RVH)

Clinical Features

In most patients with RVH, one or more of these features will be noted:

- Onset of hypertension before age 30 or after age 50

- Rapid progression of the degree of hypertension
- A diastolic bruit lateral to the midline, just below the rib cage
- Poor response to most antihypertensive drugs
- Rapid progression of renal insufficiency after use of a converting enzyme inhibitor (CEI) usually heralds bilateral renal hypertension or stenosis of the artery to a solitary kidney. In both settings, the renal circulation is critically dependent on high levels of angiotensin II (A-II) and renal blood flow is markedly reduced when A-II levels are lowered by the CEI

In the younger, particularly women, medial fibroplasia is the most common form of renal vascular disease. In the older, atherosclerotic plaques are most common.

Diagnosis

In some, renovascular hypertension cannot be distinguished on clinical grounds from primary hypertension. Nothing should be lost if the diagnosis is not made in such patients, as long as their hypertension can be well controlled and usual indices of renal function (serum creatinine) remain normal.

Those with the suggestive features listed above should be evaluated for RVH. The more suggestive the features, the more essential it is to do the definitive diagnostic test, a renal arteriogram. The use of digital subtraction equipment makes arteriography safe enough to be done as an outpatient procedure. Intravenous pyelography, peripheral blood renin levels and digital subtraction venous angiography have little place in the evaluation. Renal vein renin ratios may be useful to establish the diagnosis.

Therapy

Medical therapy, even if successful in control of hypertension, may not stop the progress of renal atrophy. Surgical repair is preferable, particularly in younger patients. Percutaneous angioplasty will likely be used increasingly as initial therapy, particularly in poor surgical candidates. It may be repeated in those who respond but in whom hypertension recurs.

References:

Anderson S, Meyer TW, Rennke HG, Brenner BM: Control of glomerular hypertension limits glomerular injury in rats with reduced renal mass. J Clin Invest 1985;76:612-619.

Luscher TF, Wanner C, Hauri D, Siegenthaler W, Vetter W: Curable renal parenchymatous hypertension: current diagnosis and management. Cardiol 1985;72(Suppl 1):33-45.

Needleman P, Greenwald JE: Atriopeptin: A cardiac hormone intimately involved in fluid, electrolyte, and blood-pressure homeostasis. N Engl J Med 1986;314:828-834.

Thind GS: Role of renal venous renins in the diagnosis and management of renovascular hypertension. J Urol 1985;134:2-5.

Vaughan ED: Renovascular hypertension. Kidney Int 1985;27:811-27.

#6 Secondary Hypertension: Adrenal

Hypertension accompanies hyperfunction of the adrenal medulla (pheochromocytoma) or cortex (Cushing's syndrome from excess cortisol or primary aldosteronism). In total, these syndromes comprise less than 1% of hypertension among adults. In children, hypersecretion of mineralocorticoids can be the consequence of congenital adrenal enzyme deficiences (congenital adrenal hyperplasia).

PHEOCHROMOCYTOMA

Approximately 80% are unilateral, benign tumors; another 10% are malignant; approximately 10% are bilateral benign tumors, often as part of the multiple endocrine adenoma (MEA) syndrome accompanied by medullary cancer of the thyroid.

Clinical Features

The hypertension may be episodic or sustained but intermittent "spells" that are almost always noted involve:

- Headache
- Tachycardia
- Sweating
- Tremor

The excess catecholamines usually induce a hypermetabolic state with:

- Weight loss
- Hyperglycemia

- Intense peripheral vasoconstriction with paleness

Diagnosis

Patients with widely fluctuating blood pressure and repeated "spells" should have a spot urine analyzed for metanephrine as a screening test. If the spot urine metanephrine is above 1.0 μg per mg creatinine, a 24 hour urine should be analyzed for metanephrine and catecholamines. Further documentation may be obtained by measurement of plasma catecholamines, first with the patient in a basal state and then 3 hours after 0.3 mg of clonidine which will suppress catecholamine secretion from normal adrenals but not from pheochromocytomas.

An abdominal CAT scan will usually demonstrate the tumor.

Therapy

Surgery should be performed after the manifestations of catecholamine excess are reversed by alpha-receptor blockade, preferably with dibenzyline or prazosin and, if tachycardia is prominent, the addition of a beta-blocker.

CUSHING'S SYNDROME

Hypertension is present in approximately 85% of patients with Cushing's syndrome whether it is caused by:

- Bilateral adrenal hyperplasia from ACTH hypersecretion from the pituitary or an ectopic tumor

- A benign adrenal tumor
- An adrenal carcinoma

Clinical Features

Cortisol excess is usually manifested by:

- Redistribution of body fat (trunkal obesity)
- Decrease in protein synthesis (thin skin with striae and ecchymoses, osteoporosis)
- Increase in glucose synthesis (hyper-glycemia)

Diagnosis

Measurement of plasma cortisol obtained the morning after a 1 mg dose of dexamethasone at bedtime is an excellent screening test, with almost all non-Cushing's patients suppressing below 7 μg/dl. Documentation of the type of Cushing's can be made by more prolonged administration of varying doses of dexamethasone, measuring 24 hour urine cortisol levels. Plasma ACTH levels and CT scans will provide additional confirmation of the type of Cushing's and may supplant the prolonged dexamethasone suppression tests.

Therapy

The source of the cortisol excess, either from the pituitary in those with bilateral hyperplasia or from an adrenal tumor, should be surgically re-moved. Various inhibitors of cortisol synthesis are available to prepare for surgery or to provide at least partial control for those in whom surgery is not feasible.

PRIMARY ALDOSTERONISM

Mineralocorticoid excess may arise from a solitary benign adenoma or bilateral hyperplasia. In general, secretion is greater from an adenoma so the manifestations are more severe:

- Plasma potassium is lower
- Plasma renin activity lower
- Plasma and urine aldosterone higher

Clinical Features

The syndrome should be considered in hypertensives with hypokalemia that is not provoked by diuretics, GI losses, etc. Almost all patients will have hypertension, which is often severe in degree, and hypokalemia, which may be intermittent (Figure 2).

Diagnosis

Urine potassium wastage of more than 30 mmol/day in the face of low plasma $K+$ should be used as a screening test (without sodium restriction or $K+$ supplementation). Autonomous hypersecretion of aldosterone may be demonstrated by failure to suppress plasma aldosterone below 6 ng/dl after 2 liters of I.V. normal saline over 4 hours. CAT scans will usually demonstrate the adrenal pathology but a number of special procedures may be needed for additional confirmation if a tumor is not seen.

Therapy

Adenomas should be surgically removed. Bilateral hyperplasia should be controlled with the aldosterone antagonist spironolactone. If that is poorly tolerated, amiloride or triamterene will usually correct the hypokalemia. A thiazide diuretic may also be needed.

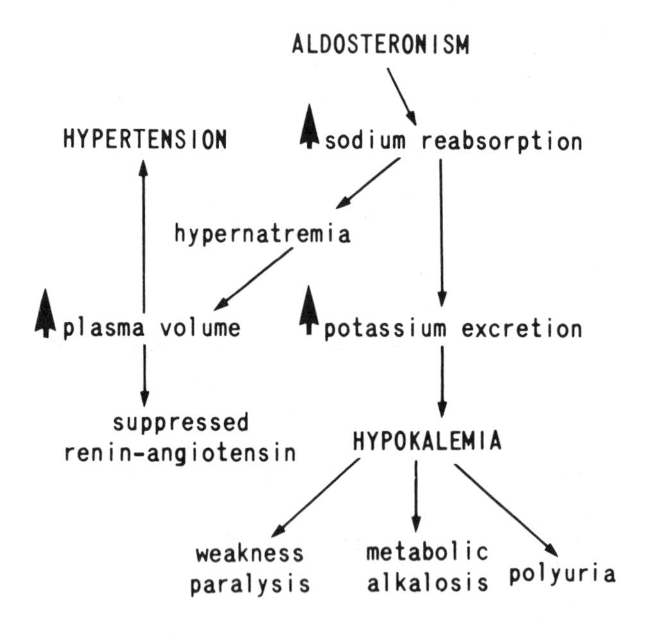

FIGURE 2. The pathophysiology of primary aldosteronism (From Kaplan NM. *Clinical Hypertension. 4th ed.,* Baltimore: Williams & Wilkins, 1986.)

References:

Biglieri EG: Rare causes of adrenocortical hypertension. Cardiol 1985;72(Suppl 1):70-5.

Chatal JF, Charbonnel B: Comparison of iodobenzylguanidine imaging with computed tomography in locating pheochromocytoma. J Clin Endocrinol Metab 1985;61:769-72.

Gifford RW, Bravo EL, Manger WM: Diagnosis and management of pheochromocytoma. Cardiol 1985;72(Suppl 1):126-130.

Kennedy L, Atkinson AB, Johnston H, Sheridan B, Hadden DR: Serum cortisol concentrations during low dose dexamethasone suppression test to screen for Cushing's syndrome. Br Med J 1984;289:1188-91.

Ross EJ, Linch DC: Cushing's syndrome - killing disease: discriminatory value of signs and symptoms aiding early diagnosis. Lancet 1982;2:646-9.

Vetter H, Fischer M, Galanski M, et al.: Primary aldosteronism: diagnosis and noninvasive lateralization procedures. Cardiol 1985;72(Suppl 1):57-63.

#7 Secondary Hypertension: Estrogen and Pregnancy

As many as 5% of women who take estrogen-containing oral contraceptives (OCs) and a somewhat smaller percentage of pregnant women will develop reversible hypertension. The former contributes to the vascular complications of OCs, the latter is a major cause of fetal mortality.

ESTROGEN-INDUCED HYPERTENSION

7.

Although the use of estrogens as postmenopausal replacement therapy does not lead to hypertension, their use in the form of oral contraceptives may do so.

Clinical Features

The blood pressure rises a few mm Hg in most who take estrogen-containing OCs. About 5% will rise beyond 140/90 within 5 years. If the OC is stopped hypertension will recede in about two-thirds of this 5%. The remaining one-third will either have underlying primary hypertension or have suffered vascular damage that sustains the OC-induced rise in blood pressure.

The hypertension is usually mild but rarely may induce severe renal vascular damage. The mechanism for the hypertension is uncertain but may involve estrogen-induced increases in renin substrate that somehow cause increased angiotensin II levels. Less hypertension may accompany the use of OCs with low doses of estrogen.

Management

Women over age 35 should not use OCs, particularly if they smoke cigarettes. When used for temporary birth control in younger women, they are quite safe. The blood pressure should be monitored every 3 to 6 months. If hypertension develops, another form of contraceptive should be substituted.

PREGNANCY HYPERTENSION

During pregnancy, hypertension may be noted early, when it usually represents primary hypertension, or late, when it usually represents the self-limited process, pregnancy-induced hypertension (PIH). The latter, if accompanied by proteinuria and edema, is usually called preeclampsia; if encephalopathy and convulsions ensue, the process is called eclampsia.

Clinical Features

In response to vasodilation, the blood pressure normally falls during the first and second trimesters, with levels of 100/60 commonly noted. Women who have unrecognized hypertension before pregnancy may lower their high levels enough to no longer be hypertensive. When their levels rise during the later months, they may be thought to have PIH, the self-limited disease that arises during the last trimester and disappears soon after delivery. Edema and proteinuria usually occur with PIH.

Mechanisms

PIH is most likely to appear among young primagravida and those with either underlying vascular disease (diabetes, primary hypertension) or large placental mass (multiple births, moles). These associations have suggested that the process is induced by reduced uteroplacental blood flow. Hemodynamically, the vascular bed is constricted. The vasoconstriction has been attributed to both increased levels of renin-angiotensin and reduced levels of vasodilatory prostaglandins, perhaps associated with an excess of thromboxanes. A reduced incidence of PIH has been reported among women considered to be susceptible who were given 60 mg a day of aspirin during the last trimester of pregnancy.

Management

PIH is diagnosed if the blood pressure rises more than 30/15 mm Hg or to a level above 140/90 in the last half of pregnancy. Levels of DBP above 85 mm Hg, particularly if accompanied by proteinuria, are associated with increased fetal mortality. Women diagnosed as having PIH should restrict activity and be carefully monitored, preferably in a high-risk pregnancy unit. Antihypertensives are given only if DBP remains above 100 mm Hg and diuretics are used only if congestive heart failure supervenes.

Women with chronic hypertension have been successfully managed with methyldopa and, more recently, beta-blockers.

If eclampsia threatens, parenteral magnesium is used. The aim of management, overall, is to allow the fetus to reach adequate maturity while protecting the mother from vascular damage.

References:

Fowler WL, Johnson JA, Kurz KD, Payne CG: Renin-angiotensin mechanisms in oral contraceptive hypertension in conscious rats. Am J Physiol 1985;248:H695-H699.

Gallery ED, Ross MR, Gyory AZ: Antihypertensive treatment in pregnancy: analysis of different responses to oxprenolol and methyldopa. Br Med J 1985;291:563-6.

Jeremy JY, Barradas MA, Mikhailidis OP, Dandona P: Placental prostacyclin production in normal and toxemic pregnancies. Am J Obstet Gynecol 1986;154:212-213.

Wallenberg HCS, Dekker GA, Makovitz JW, Rotmans P: Low-dose aspirin prevents pregnancy-induced hypertension and pre-eclampsia in angiotensin-sensitive primigravidae. Lancet 1986;1:1-3.

Ylikorkala O, Makila U-M: Prostacyclin and thromboxane in gynecology and obstetrics. Am J Obstet Gynecol 1985;152:318:29.

#8 Secondary Hypertension: Other Causes

The large number of relatively rare forms of secondary hypertension infrequently pose either diagnostic or therapeutic difficulty provided they are included in the routine evaluation process. The following covers only the more common or potentially serious forms.

HORMONAL

Hyperparathyroidism

Hypercalcemia from any cause may increase peripheral resistance and raise the blood pressure. Most patients with hyperparathyroidism are hypertensive, although the blood pressure becomes normal only in a minority after cure of the hyperparathyroidism.

Hypothyroidism

The diastolic blood pressure may be increased from peripheral vasoconstriction but the systolic level is usually not increased since cardiac output is reduced.

Hyperthyroidism

The high cardiac output tends to raise systolic levels but the diastolic is usually reduced, presumably because of peripheral vasodilation in response to increased metabolic demands.

Acromegaly

Most patients are hypertensive, likely as a result of fluid volume excess.

STRESS/SURGERY

Acute Stress and Anxiety

Marked activation of the sympathetic nervous system may induce considerable hypertension. Patients with severe chest pain from myocardial ischemia or abdominal pain from acute pancreatitis usually have significant hypertension which may rapidly recede as the pain is relieved. Caution should be taken in using potent parenteral antihypertensive agents in such patients unless their high pressures remain a threat after relief of their acute symptoms.

Transient elevations in pressure may accompany anxiety-induced acute hyperventilation.

Post-operative

Blood pressures may rise during and after surgery in response to various stimuli, including hypoxia, pain, and volume excess. A particularly high frequency of hypertension follows coronary bypass surgery, likely as a result of marked sympathetic nervous stimulation. Surgery on the carotid arteries may also be followed by significant hypertension.

Various parenteral antihypertensive agents have been used to treat peri-operative hypertension. Nitroprusside is most effective but cumbersome to use; labetalol or hydralazine, particularly with a beta-blocker, may be adequate alternatives.

Burns

Many with third-degree burns over more than 20% of body surface will develop hypertension which may require appropriate therapy.

NEUROGENIC

Sleep Apnea

As many as half of middle-aged hypertensive men may have sleep apnea, particularly if they are overweight. In most, the apnea is obstructive rather than central and therefore has been assumed to be the cause of the hypertension rather than a consequence of CNS damage. Relief of airway obstruction has been shown to result in lowering of blood pressure.

Sympathomimetic Drugs

Street drugs (amphetamines, cocaine) and over the counter drugs (phenylpropanolamine) may induce considerable hypertension.

Increased intracranial pressure

Brain tumors, acute strokes, and head trauma may cause significant hypertension, presumably by irritation of vasomotor centers or disruptions of sympathetic nervous control.

References:

Cooper TJ, Clutton-Brock TH, Jones SN, Tinker J, Treasure T: Factors relating to the development of hypertension after cardiopulmonary bypass. Br Heart J 1985;54:91-5.

Daniels J, Goodman AD: Hypertension and hyperparathyroidism: inverse relation of serum phosphate level and blood pressure. Am J Med 1983;75:17-23.

Norton PG, Dunn EV:Snoring as a risk factor for disease: an epidemiological survey. Br Med J 1985;291:630-2.

Pentel PR, Asinger RW, Benowitz NL: Propranolol antagonism of phenylpropanolamine-induced hypertension. Clin Pharmacol Ther 1985;37:488-94.

#9 Non-Drug Therapy: Dietary

Once hypertension is diagnosed and the patient evaluated, therapy should be provided. For many, therapy will include antihypertensive drugs. Issues concerning the decision to use drugs are included in Section 11 and specifics about the various agents are included in other sections. Whether or not drugs are used, a variety of non-drug therapies should be offered to all patients with any degree of hypertension. Those involving the diet will be included in this section. The remainder is included in Section 10.

WEIGHT REDUCTION

Almost half of all hypertensive people are overweight. As weight is gained, the blood pressure tends to rise; if weight is lost, the blood pressure usually falls. The mechanisms responsible are uncertain but sleep apnea may be involved in a segment of the obese hypertensive population that may be much larger than now recognized. Studies have shown that 30% or more of even slightly obese hypertensives have sleep apnea and that, at least in some, the hypertension may recede when the sleep apnea is overcome.

Calories should be restricted in a manner appropriate to the individual patient. For most, a 1200 calorie low-fat diet will provide gradual weight loss without discomfort. For some, more restrictive diets may be needed, such as the substitution of a 400 calorie per day high quality protein-powder with appropriate electrolyte and vitamin supplements.

SODIUM RESTRICTION

Restriction of dietary sodium to 2g per day (88 mmol or 5g of NaCl) will lower the blood pressure by 5 to 10 mm Hg in a significant number of "sodium-sensitive" hypertensives. This degree of restriction can be attained by avoiding highly salted foods, e.g. pickles, processed meats, sauerkraut, and adding no salt at the table or in the cooking. KCl may be used as a salt substitute, either alone or with NaCl.

An awareness is required of the "hidden" sodium present in most processed foods such as canned vegetables and many breakfast cereals (see Table 2). Fresh or unprocessed frozen foods should be used whenever possible.

Although not all patients will respond to such moderate sodium restriction, no harm should occur from the return to the natural lower-sodium diet consumed by humans throughout history until the recent past. The reduction in sodium may reduce potassium loss if diuretics are given and the lower-sodium fresh foods will likely have higher amounts of potassium than are present in their processed forms.

More rigid sodium restriction may be needed for patients with renal failure or severe heart failure. If needed, low-sodium preparations of a number of processed foods are available.

Potassium Supplementation

Correction of hypokalemia may lower the blood pressure. However, there is no reason for additional potassium to be given to normokalemic patients, particularly if they follow a 2g sodium diet which will likely have a fairly high potassium content. Supplements of KCl may be required to replenish potassium deficiency since dietary sources of potassium may be largely accompanied by non-reabsorbable anions which reduce retention of the potassium.

Calcium Supplementation

In a few studies, use of 1 to 2g per day of calcium has been found to lower blood pressure and some hypertensives, particularly elderly women, may ingest less calcium than recommended for prevention of osteoporosis.

Magnesium Supplementation

Patients receiving diuretics may become magnesium depleted. Magnesium supplements were shown in one study, but not in another, to lower blood pressure. It may not be possible to replete potassium deficiency with KCl in the presence of magnesium deficiency.

Other Dietary Changes

A few well-controlled studies have shown that the intake of a lower saturated, higher unsaturated fat diet will reduce the blood pressure. The effect may be attributable to an increase in synthesis of vasodilatory prostaglandins.

One study has shown a fall in blood pressure with a high fiber diet.

Moderation of Alcohol

Besides adding calories, alcohol consumption may raise the blood pressure. In large population surveys, daily consumption of more than 2 ounces of alcohol per day is associated with higher blood pressure and more than 3 ounces per day is often associated with overt hypertension. One ounce per day, i.e. 2 beers, 2 glasses of wine or 2 mixed drinks, will likely not raise the blood pressure but will provide protection against coronary disease and mortality. This has been demonstrated in many epidemiological surveys wherein those who drink 1 to 2 ounces of ethanol per day have less CHD than do those who do not drink ethanol.

TABLE 2
THE SODIUM CONTENT OF SOME AMERICAN FOODS

(1000 mg Sodium = 44 mEq Sodium)

Comparable foods with either low or high sodium content

Low

Shredded Wheat:	1 mg/oz
Green Beans, fresh:	5 mg/cup
Orange Juice:	2 mg/cup
Turkey, roasted:	70 mg/3-oz
Ground Beef:	57 mg/3-oz
Pork, uncooked:	65 mg/3-oz

High

Corn Flakes:	305 mg/oz
Green Beans, canned:	925 mg/cup
Tomato Juice:	640 mg/cup
Turkey dinner:	1,735 mg
Frankfurter, beef:	425 mg each
Bacon, uncooked:	1,400 mg/3-oz

Sodium content of some "Fast Foods"

Kentucky Fried Chicken (three pieces of chicken, potatoes, gravy, cole slaw and roll)	2,285 mg
McDonald's Big Mac	962 mg
Burger King Whopper	909 mg
Dairy Queen Chili Dog	939 mg
Taco Bell Enchirito	1,175 mg

Some foods with very high sodium content

Catsup, one tablespoon:	156 mg
Olive, one:	165 mg
Cinnamon roll, one:	630 mg
Soup (chicken noodle), one cup:	1,050 mg
Dill pickle, one large:	1,928 mg

References:

Cappuccio FP, Markandu ND, Beynon GW, Shore AC, Sampson B, MacGregor GA: Lack of effect of oral magnesium on high blood pressure: a double blind study. Br Med J 1985;291:235-8.

Kaplan NM: Non-drug treatment of hypertension. Ann Intern Med 1985;102:359-73.

Kaplan NM, Carnegie A, Raskin P, Heller JA, Simmons M: Potassium supplementation in hypertensive patients with diuretic-induced hypokalemia. N Engl J Med 1985;312:746-9.

MacMahon SW, Wileken DEL, Macdonald GJ: The effect of weight reduction on left ventricular mass. N Engl J Med 1986;314:334-9.

Malhotra H, Mehta SR, Mathur D, Khandelwal PD: Pressor effects of alcohol in normotensive and hypertensive subjects. Lancet 1985;2:584-6.

McCarron DA, Morris CD: Blood pressure response to oral calcium in persons with mild or moderate hypertension. Ann Intern Med 1985;103:825-31.

Truswell AS: Diet and Hypertension. Br Med J 1985;291:125-6

Notes

#10 Non-Drug Therapy: Other

Beyond dietary changes, other non-drug therapies may help lower the blood pressure. These include isotonic exercise and one or another form of relaxation therapy. Claims have been made for other modalities as varied as garlic and acupuncture but their efficacy has not been shown in properly controlled clinical trials.

ISOTONIC EXERCISE

A number of studies have shown that regular isotonic (dynamic or aerobic) exercise is accompanied by a fall in blood pressure. Few of these studies have been well controlled and some of the antihypertensive effects of exercise may reflect coincidental weight loss, changes in diet, etc. Regardless, hypertensives should be encouraged to perform regular isotonic exercises, if they enjoy doing them.

The form of exercise is irrelevant as long as it is isotonic, i.e. involves active movement of muscles. During isotonic exercise, cardiac output rises but peripheral resistance falls from vasodilation in muscle vasculature. Systolic blood pressure rises but diastolic pressure tends to fall or remain the same. Isometric exercise, i.e. increased tension without movement, is associated with a reflex increase in both cardiac output and peripheral resistance, causing marked rises in both systolic and diastolic blood pressure while the isometric exercise is being performed.

Stress Tests

Some normotensive people have marked increases in systolic blood pressure, beyond 180 mm Hg, during the intense exercise of a stress test. Preliminary data suggests that such people may have a somewhat higher likelihood of subsequently developing permanent hypertension.

Amount of Exercise

To reach the "conditioned" state of cardiac performance, 20 to 30 minutes of sustained exercise at 70% of maximal capacity, usually determined from the rise in pulse rate, is required 3 times each week. The level of exercise that accomplishes the greatest fall in blood pressure has not been determined.

RELAXATION THERAPY

Almost all forms of relaxation therapy have been said to lower the blood pressure. These include:

- Progressive muscle relaxation
- Yoga
- Biofeedback
- Transcendental meditation
- The Chinese breathing exercise Qi Gong
- Hypnosis

A few controlled studies have shown a sustained effect beyond the duration of the relaxation procedure. Those patients who are willing to continue the practice of one or another relaxation therapy should be encouraged to do so.

AN OVERALL NON-DRUG PROGRAM

An overall non-drug program includes:

- Reduce excess body weight by caloric restriction. Caution against the use of over-the-counter appetite suppressants — most contain the sympathomimetic phenylpropanolamine which may raise the blood pressure.
- Restrict dietary sodium to 2g per day (88 mmol or 5g of NaCl), about half the amount in the usual American diet.
- Reduce dietary saturated fat and cholesterol.
- Maintain adequate intake of potassium, calcium and magnesium, supplementing those who are deficient.
- Limit alcohol intake to no more than 2 ounces and preferably one ounce per day (one ounce of alcohol contained in 2 usual portions of beer, wine or spirits).
- Perform 20 to 30 minutes of isotonic exercise at least 3 times a week.
- Use whatever form of relaxation therapy that is acceptable.
- Stop smoking. This will likely not influence the blood pressure but will have a powerfully beneficial effect on overall cardiovascular health.

References:

Cade R, Mars D, Wagemaker H, et al.: Effect of aerobic exercise training on patients with systemic arterial hypertension. Am J Med 1984;77:785-90.

Cottier C, Shapiro K, Julius S: Treatment of mild hypertension with progressive muscle relaxation. Arch Intern Med 1984;144:1954-8.

Duncan JJ, Farr JE, Upton SJ, et al: The effects of aerobic exercise on plasma catecholamines and blood pressure in patients with mild essential hypertension. JAMA 1985;254:2609-13.

Health and Public Policy Committee: Biofeedback for hypertension. Ann Intern Med 1985;102:709-15.

Jennings G, Nelson L, Nestel P, et al: The effects of changes in physical activity on major cardiovascular risk factors, hemodynamics, sympathetic function, and glucose utilization in man. Circulation 1986;73:30-40.

Kannel WB, Wilson P, Blair SN: Epidemiological assessment of the role of physical activity and fitness in development of cardiovascular disease. Am Heart J l985;109:876-85.

Stamler R, Stamler J, Grimm R, et al: Nonpharmalogical control of hypertension. Preventive Med 1985;14:336-45.

#11 The Decision to Use Drugs

Patients with uncomplicated mild hypertension, defined as DBP between 90 and 104 mm Hg, who comprise by far the largest portion of the population with an elevated blood pressure, need not immediately be started on antihypertensive drugs. Although immediate start of therapy has become common practice, a more conservative approach is recommended for the following reasons:

First, such patients are at little short-term risk and will not be endangered by postponement of drug therapy until the permanence of their hypertension is ascertained and non-drug therapies are given a chance to lower the DBP to below 90 mm Hg.

Second, many of these patients will have a persistently lower blood pressure after 2 to 3 months of repeated measurements. However, if they become normotensive, they should remain under surveillance since they are more likely to become hypertensive in the future.

Third, non-drug therapies may bring and keep their pressures down.

Fourth, and most importantly, all drug therapies have risks, costs, and side effects. Though these may be minimized, they cannot be completely avoided. Often the risks of not using them clearly outweighs the risks of their use — as in patients with high overall cardiovascular risk, significant target organ damage or DBP that averages above 100 mm Hg. But many with DBP below 95 can safely be managed without drugs and many authorities, particularly outside the United

States, advise that drugs be given only if the DBP remains above 100 mg Hg. The 1984 report of the Joint National Committee advises drug therapy for all with DBP above 95 and for higher risk patients with DBP between 90 and 94.

THE ISSUE OF PROTECTION

Despite their risks, drugs would be indicated for more patients if there were clear evidence that they protect against major cardiovascular morbidity and mortality. A number of large clinical trials completed from 1978 through 1985 have demonstrated protection against stroke. But protection against coronary disease, the most frequent and serious complication associated with hypertension has not been clearly shown. In fact, higher rates of coronary mortality were noted among the treated patients in some of the trials.

The failure to demonstrate protection against coronary disease in these trials may reflect the manner by which the pressure was lowered. In most, large doses of diuretics were the first and often the only drug used.Diuretic-induced hypokalemia may have been responsible for higher rates of sudden (coronary) death.

The only trial to date that has examined two different drug therapies, a diuretic and a beta-blocker, performed by the Medical Research Council of England, failed to find a clear advantage from either. In that trial only those men who did not smoke were protected against coronary disease by the beta-blocker whereas the diuretic was better in protecting against stroke.

THE ISSUE OF SIDE EFFECTS

In most of the large clinical trials, from 20 to 40% of patients started on drug therapy stopped it, in about half because of adverse reactions. Even more than this percentage will have one or another side effect. Although most of these are mild and often only transient, they can and do interfere with the quality of life. Some, such as mental dullness, may be so subtle as to be inapparent to the patient (although often apparent to those around him). Others, such as impotence, may not be discussed or related to the drug. The inability to gain erection may be a non-specific effect of any and all antihypertensives, which by successfully lowering blood pressure may lower blood flow into the genital vessels, particularly in those with underlying atherosclerotic vascular disease (see Section 28).

The decision to start drug therapy, then, should not be taken lightly but made with careful consideration of the implications involved. Reasonable certainty should exist that the benefits will outweigh the risks and side effects.

References:

Anonymous: Treatment of hypertension: the 1985 results (Editorial). Lancet 1985;2:645-7.

Brett AS: Ethical issues in risk factor intervention. Am J Med 1984;76:557-61.

Cloher TP, Whelton PK: Physician approach to the recognition and initial management of hypertension. Arch Intern Med 1986;146:529-33.

Hyman D, Kaplan NM: Treatment of patients with mild hypertension (Editorial). Hypertension 1985;7:165-70.

Kuller LH, Hulley S, Cohen JD, Neaton J: Unexpected effects of treating hypertension in men with electrocardiographic abnormalities: a critical analysis. Circulation 1986;73:114-23.

Logan AG: Report of the Canadian Hypertension Society's consensus conference on the management of mild hypertension. Can Med Assoc J 1984;131:1053-7.

Medical Research Council Working Party: MRC trial of treatment of mild hypertension: principal results. Br Med J 1985;291:97-104.

Moser M: The case for treating mild hypertension. J Cardiovasc Pharmacol 1985;7:S102-S108.

Sleight P: High blood pressure: what level to treat? J Cardiovasc Pharmacol 1985;7:S109-S111.

#12 General Guidelines for Drug Therapy

As many as half of patients begun on antihypertensive therapy will not be taking it one year later, most of them simply stopping the medication because of inadequate followup, lack of perceived benefit or side effects. Care must be taken to prescribe drugs in a way which can easily be remembered by asymptomatic people, which will interfere little with various activities, and which will cause few side effects. These guidelines should help improve patient compliance to therapy:

- Establish the goal of therapy — to reduce blood pressure to normotensive levels with minimal or no side effects.
- Educate the patient about his disease and its treatment.
- Maintain contact with the patient.
  - Encourage visits and calls to allied health personnel.
  - Allow the pharmacist to monitor therapy.
  - Make contact with patients who do not return.
- Keep care inexpensive and simple.
  - Do the least work-up needed to rule out secondary causes.
  - Obtain follow-up laboratory data only yearly unless indicated more often.
  - Use home blood pressure readings.
  - Use non-drug, no cost therapies.
  - Use the fewest daily doses of drugs needed.
  - If appropriate, use combination tablets.

- Prescribe according to pharmacological principles.
  - Add one drug at a time.
  - Start with small doses, aiming for 5 to 10 mm Hg reductions at each step.
  - Prevent volume overload with adequate diuretic and sodium restriction.
  - Stop unsuccessful therapy and try a different approach.
  - If therapy is only partially successful, additional drugs of different classes may be added, preferably one at a time, in sufficient doses to achieve the goal of therapy.
  - Anticipate side effects.
  - Adjust therapy to ameliorate side effects that do not spontaneously disappear.
- Be aware of the problem and be alert to signs of patient nonadherence. Have the patient bring medications to the office so that pill counts and checks on numbers of refills can be done if the blood pressure has not responded.

The management of resistant hypertension is presented in Section 29.

References:

Eraker SA, Kirscht JP, Becker MH: Understanding and improving patient compliance. Ann Intern Med 1984;100:258-68.

Greenfield S, Kaplan S, Ware JE: Expanding patient involvement in care: effects on patient outcomes. Ann Intern Med 1985;102:520-8.

Zismer DK, Gillum RF, Johnson A, Becerra J, Johnson TH: Improving hypertension control in a private medical practice. Arch Intern Med 1982;142:297-9.

#13 Diuretics: Thiazides

The moderately long acting diuretic hydrochlorothiazide is the most popular drug in the United States for therapy of hypertension. Although it may become less commonly chosen as the initial drug, hydrochlorothiazide or other thiazide diuretics will almost certainly continue to be widely used. Loop diuretics and potassium-saving agents are considered in Section 14.

TABLE 3
CHARACTERISTICS OF DIURETICS

	Daily Dosage (mg)	Duration of Action (hrs)
Thiazides		
Bendroflumethiazide (Naturetin)	2.5-5.0	More than 18
Benzthiazide (Aquatag, Exna)	12.5-50	12-18
Chlorothiazide (Diuril)	250-500	6-12
Cyclothiazide (Anhydron)	1-2	18-24
Hydrochlorothiazide (Esidrix, HydroDiuril, Oretic)	12.5-50	12-18
Hydroflumethiazide (Saluron)	12.5-50	18-24
Methyclothiazide (Enduron)	2.5-5.0	More than 24
Polythiazide (Renese)	1-4	24-48
Trichlormethiazide (Metahydrin, Naqua)	1-4	More than 24
Related sulfonamide compounds		
Chlorthalidone (Hygroton)	12.5-50	24-72
Indapamide (Lozol)	2.5	24
Metolazone (Zaroxolyn, Diulo)	1.0-5.0	24
Quinethazone (Hydromox)	50-100	18-24
Loop diuretics		
Bumetanide (Bumex)	1-10	4-6
Ethacrynic acid (Edecrin)	50-200	12
Furosemide (Lasix)	40-480	4-6
Potassium-sparing agents		
Amiloride (Midamor)	5-10	24
Spironolactone (Aldactone)	25-100	8-12
Triamterene (Dyrenium)	50-100	12

Types

Thiazides are sulfonamide derivatives which cause as much as 5 to 8% of the filtered sodium load to be excreted by blocking reabsorption in the early distal tubule at the cortical diluting segment. They differ in duration of action, which in turn can alter the degree of metabolic side effects. Since the mode of action and potency are similar, they share the same types of side effects.

Chemical additions to the thiazide structure provide chlorthalidone (Hygroton) with more prolonged action and indapamide (Lozol) with some additional effects on peripheral resistance.

Metalozone (Diulo, Zaroxolyn) also has effects within the proximal tubule so it is a more potent diuretic which will work even in the presence of significant renal insufficiency.

Mode of Action

To lower the blood pressure, diuretics must initially induce a natriuresis which shrinks blood volume. This activates various mechanisms responsible for maintenance of fluid volume, particularly the renin-angiotensin-aldosterone system. These, in turn, limit the degree of volume depletion.

At the same time, continued diuretic use leads to a fall in peripheral vascular resistance which is the major reason for the continued antihypertensive effect.

Most patients will achieve a 10 mm Hg fall in blood pressure with daily diuretic therapy. Those with more "volume dependent" hypertension, as demonstrable by lower levels of plasma renin activity, tend to respond particularly well. These include many black and elderly hypertensives.

Doses

Thiazides have a fairly flat dose-response curve, so that most of the antihypertensive effect is achieved with low doses (Figure 3). Even though as much as 200 mg of hydrochlorothiazide per day has been used in the past, as little as 25 mg given once a day will provide most of the blood pressure lowering effect and less of the metabolic side effects of larger doses. When added to other drugs, as little as 12.5 mg may be effective.

Despite having only a 12 to 16 hour duration of action, a single morning dose of hydrochlorothiazide will provide sustained antihypertensive effect, while reducing potassium wastage during the nighttime.

Causes for Resistance

If an inadequate response is observed with 25 mg of hydrochlorothiazide, the dose can be increased to 50 mg or more although little additional antihypertensive effect usually is seen above 50 mg per day. The poor response may reflect either an overwhelming load of dietary sodium or an impaired renal capacity to excrete the sodium. Patients with serum creatinine above 2.5 mg/dl likely will not respond to thiazides.

Overly vigorous diuretic therapy may activate the renin-angiotensin-aldosterone mechanism excessively. Thereby the antihypertensive effect of the diuretic may be antagonized by the vasoconstrictive effect of angiotensin and potassium wastage may be increased by the aldosterone-mediated exchange of more potassium for sodium.

When more severe hypertensives are given progressively more therapy —particularly if it includes a vasodilator — the reduction in blood pressure may lead to more intense sodium retention, mandating the use of additional diuretic. This has been noted particularly with the use of minoxidil, even more so when it is given to patients with renal insufficiency.

SIDE EFFECTS

A number of side effects accompany the use of diuretics. Some are allergic or idiosyncratic, such as skin rash and pancreatitis. More common are a variety of biochemical changes, which in large part reflect an exaggeration of the expected, desired effects of the drugs (Figure 4). Though their manifestations may not be clinically obvious, they pose more serious potential hazards over the long duration for which these drugs may be used.

HYPOKALEMIA

Urine potassium wastage is inevitable with diuretic therapy. By blocking reabsorption of sodium chloride in the distal tubule, the diuretic causes additional tubular fluid containing sodium to be delivered to the lower portion of the nephron wherein potassium exchange for sodium occurs. The largest amount of potassium wastage occurs initially while the diuresis is maximal, but it may continue as long as the renin-aldosterone system is activated and sodium is delivered to the collecting duct.

The average fall in plasma potassium with continuous daily diuretic therapy for 4 weeks or longer is 0.7 mmol/L. Depending upon the pretreatment $K+$ level, such a fall may induce hypokalemia in approximately one-third of patients, when hypokalemia is defined as a plasma $K+$ below 3.2 mmol/L (or serum $K+$ below 3.5). The degree of fall in plasma $K+$ may be greater than the fall in intracellular potassium content.

Hypokalemia rarely causes symptoms, although muscular weakness and leg cramps may be noted. However, an increase in ventricular ectopic activity has been observed and this may be responsible for the excess rates of sudden death observed in some of the large clinical trials wherein diuretic-induced hypokalemia was frequently noted and often not treated.

Hypokalemia may also be responsible for diuretic-induced glucose intolerance and hypercholesterolemia.

Diuretic-induced hypokalemia can be minimized by these steps:

- Use the smallest dose of diuretic possible
- Use moderately long-acting diuretics such as hydrochlorothiazide rather than longer acting ones
- Reduce dietary sodium intake to 2 g (88 mmol) per day
- Increase dietary potassium intake
- Combine potassium-sparers with the diuretic (see Section 14)
- Use drugs that suppress the renin system, e.g. beta-blockers, converting enzyme inhibitors

HYPERCHOLESTEROLEMIA

A 10-20mg/dl increase in total serum cholesterol may develop and persist for years unless countered by reduction of saturated fat in the diet. The atherogenic potential of diuretic-induced rises in serum cholesterol has not been proved but probably is similar to "naturally" occuring hypercholesterolemia.

GLUCOSE INTOLERANCE

Fasting and post-prandial blood sugars may rise but overt hyperglycemia is rare, even in patients with pre-existing diabetes. A decrease in either insulin secretion or action secondary to hypokalemia may be responsible.

HYPERURICEMIA

Increased tubular reabsorption of uric acid accompanies the shrinkage of fluid volume. Diuretic-induced hyperuricemia need not be treated even if plasma levels rise above 10 mg/dl, unless gout occurs. If therapy is needed, the uricosuric agent, probenecid, is appropriate.

HYPERCALCEMIA

More calcium is reabsorbed in a manner similar to uric acid, usually raising serum calcium levels by less than 0.5 mg/dl. Overt hypercalcemia may occur in patients with pre-existing, unrecognized hyperparathyroidism.

HYPONATREMIA

A significant fall in plasma sodium is rarely noted, usually in elderly patients who are overdiuresed.

HYPOMAGNESEMIA

Magnesium wastage may accompany potassium wastage and hypomagnesemia occassionally develops.

Despite this long list of potential problems, diuretics have proven to be effective and generally safe when used in the lowest dose needed and with proper surveillance of biochemical changes.

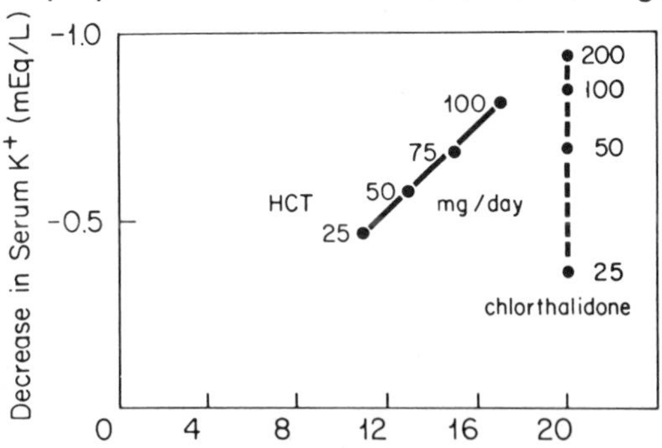

FIGURE 3. The effects of various doses of hydrochlorothiazide (HCT) and chlorthalidone on the blood pressure and serum potassium in two groups of hypertensives. The different doses of chlorthalidone and HCT were given for 6- to 8-week periods in random order. (Data on HCT taken from Degnbol et al.: Acta Med Scand 1973;193:407; data on chlorthalidone from Tweeddale et al.: Clin Pharmacol Ther 1977;22:519.)

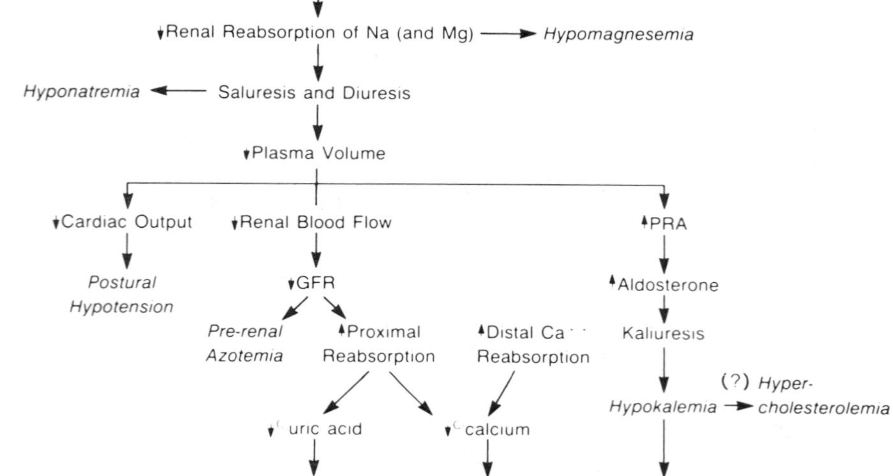

FIGURE 4. A pathogenetic scheme for the various side effects of diuretics. (From Kaplan NM. *Clinical Hypertension. 4th ed.* Baltimore: Williams & Wilkins, 1986.)

References:

Bengtsson C, Blohme G, Lapidus L, et al.: Do antihypertensive drugs precipitate diabetes? Br Med J 1984;289:1495-7.

Bennett WM, Porter GA: Efficacy and safety of metolazone in renal failure and the nephrotic syndrome. J Clin Pharmacol 1973;13:357-64.

Brand FN, McGee DL, Kannel WB, Stokes J III, Castelli WP: Hyperuricemia as a risk factor of coronary heart disease: the Framingham Study. Am J Epidemiol. 1985;121:11-18.

Freis ED: Advantages of diuretics. Am J Med 1984;77:107-9.

Jamieson MJ: Hyponatraemia. Br Med J 1985;290:1723-8.

Kaplan NM: Our appropriate concern about hypokalemia . Am J Med 1984;77:1-4.

Knochel JP: Diuretic-induced hypokalemia. Am J Med 1984;77:18-27

Lant A: Diuretics: clinical pharmacology and therapeutic use (part I). Drugs 1985;29:57-87.

Lant A: Diuretics: clinical pharmacology and therapeutic use (part II). Drugs 1985;29:162-88.

MacGregor GA, Banks RA, Markandu ND, Bayliss J, Roulston J: Lack of effect of beta-blocker on flat dose response to thiazide in hypertension: efficacy of low dose thiazide combined with beta-blocker. Br Med J 1983;286:1535-8.

Whang R, Flink EB, Dyckner T, Wester PO, Aikawa JK, Ryan MP: Magnesium depletion as a cause of refractory potassium repletion. Arch Intern Med 1985;145:1686-9.

Weidmann P, Uehlinger DE, Gerber A: Antihypertensive treatment and serum lipoproteins (Editorial Review). J Hypertension 1985;3:297-306.

#14 Diuretics: Loop and K+ Sparers

Some hypertensives may require more potent diuretics than thiazides. Those who receive a thiazide may be protected from potassium wastage by the concomitant use of a potassium-sparing agent.

LOOP DIURETICS

These agents may exert a maximal natriuretic effect of 20% of the filtered load, some 3 to 4 times more than the thiazide diuretics, by blocking sodium chloride reabsorption in the thick ascending limb of the loop of Henle. They must enter the tubular fluid to work. Therefore when renal blood flow is reduced, larger doses are needed. Their entry into the tubule may be competitively blocked by organic acids and drugs such as probenecid.

The two agents now available, furosemide (Lasix) and bumetanide (Bumex), are short acting with their effect lasting 3 to 6 hours. They must be given twice or 3 times a day to maintain the slight shrinkage of plasma volume needed to keep the blood pressure down. Therefore, they are primarily indicated for patients with reduced renal function (serum creatinine above 2.5 mg/dl) wherein thiazides are ineffectual or there is a need for more potent diuretics as with minoxidil therapy.

Side effects are similar to those seen with thiazides with the exception of hypercalcemia. They will cause less severe biochemical changes because of shorter duration of action.

Another loop diuretic, ethacrynic acid (Edecrin) is little used because of its greater ototoxicity.

POTASSIUM-SPARING AGENTS

Three are now available, one an aldosterone antagonist, the other two inhibitors of tubular K+ secretion. They are helpful in:

- Reducing thiazide-induced K+ wastage
- Specifically treating hyperaldosteronism

Spironolactone (Aldactone) + HCT = Aldactazide

This agent competitively blocks the uptake of aldosterone by its receptors, thereby antagonizing its actions. It will reduce diuretic-induced K+ loss. However, its major use is in treatment of states of aldosterone excess, whether primary or secondary, e.g. cirrhosis with ascites. Only 25-50 mg a day is needed for reduction in K+ loss but more may be needed to block hyperaldosteronism.

Side effects include:

- Capacity to induce hyperkalemia
- May interfere with testosterone synthesis, leading to impotence and gynecomastia in men and mastodynia in women

Triamterene (Dyrenium) + HCT = Dyazide or Maxzide

This is the K+ sparer contained in combination with 25 mg of hydrochlorothiazide and sold in the United States as Dyazide. The formulation, though only 30 to 40% absorbed, has been widely used on a one a day schedule, demonstrating that as little as 10 mg of hydrochlorothiazide can provide antihypertensive effect.

Recently a better absorbed formulation of triamterene plus hydrochlorothiazide has been marketed as Maxzide. Each tablet contains 50 mg of HCT, which is more diuretic than many need. One-half of a tablet per day should be adequate for most patients.

Side effects are rare. Hyperkalemia is rarely seen except in patients with renal insufficiency who are also given potassium. Renal tubular damage and renal stones have been reported.

Amiloride (Midamor) + HCT = Moduretic

This K+ sparer is chemically distinct and acts differently than triamterene. However, the effects of the two agents are quite similar. They both have limited natriuretic effect but inhibit K+ secretion in the collecting duct. It also has 50 mg of HCT and one-half of a tablet may be adequate for most patients.

References:

Andersson P-O, H-Andersen H, Hagman A, Henning R: Potassium sparing by amiloride during thiazide therapy in hypertension. Clin Pharmacol Ther 1984;36:197-200.

Keeton GR, Morrison S: Effects of frusemide in chronic renal failure. Nephron 1981;28:169-73.

Spence JD, Wong DG, Lindsay RM: Effects of triamterene and amiloride on urinary sediment in hypertensive patients taking hydrochlorothiazide. Lancet 1985;2:73-5.

Wollam GL, Tarazi RC, Bravo EL, Dustan HP: Diuretic potency of combined hydrochlorothiazide and furosemide therapy in patients with azotemia. Am J Med 1982;72:929-37.

#15 Adrenergic Inhibitors - Peripheral

The second major class of drugs are those which inhibit the activity of the adrenergic (sympathetic) nervous system. As shown in Table 4, the primary sites of action vary from the brain to the peripheral neurons. Some act as competitive inhibitors of alpha-receptors and others as blockers of beta-receptors.

The peripheral-acting agents are shown to include reserpine, which acts in the central nervous system (CNS) as well as upon peripheral neurons. These drugs are among the longest used antihypertensives, but have lost much popularity as other agents have become available. Reserpine remains an effective, generally safe, inexpensive, once-a-day drug that many find works well, particularly in combination with a diuretic.

RESERPINE (SERPASIL)

This ingredient of Indian snakeroot acts by decreasing the transport of norepinephrine into its storage granules within the adrenergic nerve endings, thereby depleting the amount of the neurotransmitter available when the nerves are stimulated.

Small amounts are effective. When used with a diuretic, as little as 0.05 mg a day may be adequate. Larger doses of 0.25 mg are frequently used, either alone or in combination. Side effects include:

- Nasal stuffiness
- Sedation
- Mental depression

These side effects are less when using smaller doses. Patients receiving the drug should be forewarned about the symptoms of depression. Claims that reserpine use was associated with an increased risk of breast cancer have not been documented and have been attributed to bias introduced by selected exclusion of certain patients from the original studies.

GUANETHIDINE (ISMELIN)

This was a popular agent since it could be used once a day in patients with all degrees of hypertension and caused no CNS side effects. The drug causes profound inhibition of peripheral sympathetic nervous activity by blocking the exit of norepinephrine from its storage granules, frequently leading to:

- Postural hypotension
- Diarrhea
- Failure of ejaculation

Although it can be well tolerated with careful titration and avoidance of rapid postural changes, the drug has largely been relegated to a last-option status.

GUANADREL (HYLOREL)

This guanethidine-like agent is easier to use because of its shorter duration of action, with less sustained interference with peripheral adrenergic action. Side effects are similar but less common. The antihypertensive efficacy is comparable to that of methyldopa.

References:

Finnerty FA, Brogden RN: Guanadrel: a review of its pharmacodynamic and pharmacokinetic properties and therapeutic use in hypertension. Drugs 1985;30:22-31.

Horwitz RI, Feinstein AR: Exclusion bias and the false relationship of reserpine and breast cancer. Arch Intern Med 1985;145:1873-5.

TABLE 4
CHARACTERISTICS OF ADRENERGIC INHIBITORS

Drug	Trade Name	Dose Range (mg/day)	Side Effects
Peripheral:			
Reserpine	Serpasil	0.05-0.25	Sedation, nasal congestion, depression
Guanethidine	Ismelin	10-150	Orthostatic hypotension, diarrhea
Guanadrel	Hylorel	10-75	Orthostatic hypotension
Central:			
Methyldopa	Aldomet	500-3000	Sedation, liver dysfunction, fever, "auto-immune" disorders
Clonidine	Catapres	0.2-1.2	Sedation, dry mouth, "withdrawal hypertension"
Guanabenz	Wytensin	8-32	Sedation, dry mouth, dizziness
Alpha-blocker:			
Prazosin	Minipress	2-20	Postural hypotention (mainly with first dose), lassitude

Beta-blockers:			
Acebutolol	Sectral	200-800	Serious: bronchospasm, congestive heart failure, masking of insulin-induced hypoglycemia, depression
Atenolol	Tenormin	25-100	
Metoprolol	Lopressor	50-300	
Nadolol	Corgard	42-320	
Pindolol	Visken	10-60	Less Serious: poor peripheral circulation, insomnia, bradycardia, fatigue, decreased exercise tolerance, hypertriglyceridemia, decrease HDL
Propranolol	Inderal	40-480	
Timolol	Blocadren	20-60	
Combined α- ***and*** β-***Blocker***			
Labetalol	Normodyne, Trandate	200-1200	Postural hypotension, beta-blocking side effects

#16 Adrenergic Inhibitors — Central Agonists

The members of this group of drugs act as alpha$_2$-receptor agonists, primarily on vasomotor centers within the brain, thereby decreasing the sympathetic outflow from the CNS (Figure 5). As a result, cardiac output is decreased slightly but the main hemodynamic effect is a fall in peripheral vascular resistance. Although the 3 currently available members of this group differ in some ways, they share a common mechanism of action and side effects. Methyldopa, however, has some unique "auto-immune" side effects.

METHYLDOPA (ALDOMET)

The most popular drug after thiazide diuretics, methyldopa is being used less since beta-blockers and a steadily increasing list of newer agents have become available.

Mechanism of Action

Methyldopa is converted into α-methylnorepinephrine which acts as an agonist (stimulant) of the central alpha-receptors. This central agonist action leads to a decrease in discharge from central vasomotor centers, dampening sympathetic nervous activity throughout the body. Blood pressure falls mainly from a decrease in peripheral resistance.

Dosage

To reduce the impact of the centrally-mediated side effects — sedation and dry mouth in particular — the initial dose should be no more than 250 mg twice a day. The total dosage can be raised to 3 g/day, however, 1 g twice a day will do almost all that is possible with the drug. One dose a day may provide 24 hour control for some, but twice a day, i.e. every 12 hours, dosage is more effective for most.

Side Effects

Beyond the common sedation and dry mouth, many experience a more subtle decrease in mental alertness. These side effects are common to all three central alpha-agonists. Methyldopa, however, induces a number of "auto-immune" disorders:

- Positive Coombs tests in as many as 25% but hemolytic anemia in very few
- Abnormal liver function tests in 8%
- Severe hepatic necrosis in a small number
- Virtually every other organ has been attacked, though the frequency is quite low

These immune-inflammatory processes are not seen with the other central agonists which are equal in effectiveness. Therefore, continued widespread use of methyldopa is difficult to justify and must be attributed to hard-to-change prescribing habits. However, patients who seem to be doing well and deny all side effects may continue to use the drug.

CLONIDINE (CATAPRES)

This drug, similar to methyldopa, differs in two important ways:

- Its duration of action is shorter
- Its dosage is smaller

The starting dose should be 0.1 mg twice a day. The shorter duration of action helps explain the somewhat higher incidence of rebound hypertension. When the drug is abruptly stopped, sympathetic nervous activity may rather quickly bounce back from its suppressed state and may overshoot. This problem is infrequent when the total dosage is kept below 0.8 mg/day. The second difference has been taken advantage of by placing the small quantity of drug needed to exert an antihypertensive effect into a patch for transdermal absorption thereby providing up to 7 days of therapy. Local skin reactions may preclude its use in 20% or more. However, the patch may provide smoother control of hypertension with fewer side effects.

GUANABENZ (WYTENSIN)

A recently introduced alpha-agonist, this drug is the most attractive of this class for these two reasons:

- It has been shown to lower total serum cholesterol levels by 5 to 10%, unlike diuretics which tend to raise cholesterol
- It has been found to cause little reactive fluid retention, so that a diuretic may not be needed to preserve its effect

The drug mimics the mode of action and side effects of clonidine in some ways. Starting dosage should be 4 mg twice a day and the maximum dosage can reach a total of 64 mg/day.

This class of drugs seems particularly attractive for those who:

- Can tolerate or escape their sedative action
- Would likely not do well with beta-blockers or diuretics

These include:

- Elderly patients
- Diabetics
- Hypercholesterolemics
- Those with asthma
- Those having peripheral vascular disease

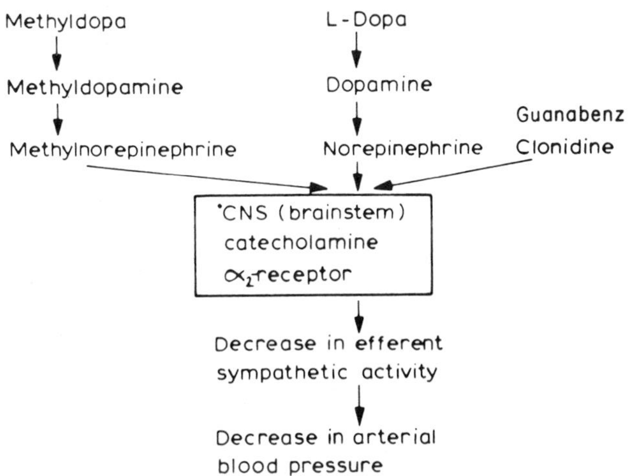

FIGURE 5. Schematic representation of the common mechanism underlying the hypotensive actions of methyldopa, clonidine and guanabenz. (From Henning M. In van Zwieten PA (ed). *Handbook of Hypertension Vo. 3,* Amsterdam: Elsevier Science Publishers, 1984.)

References:

Gehr M, MacCarthy EP, Goldberg M: Natriuretic and water diuretic effects of central α_2-adrenoceptor agonists. J Cardiovasc Pharmacol 1984;6:S781-S786.

Holmes B, Brogden RN, Heel RC, Speight TM, Avery GS: Guanabenz: a review of its pharmacodynamic properties and therapeutic efficacy in hypertension. Drugs 1983;26:212-29.

Kaplan NM: Effects of guanabenz on plasma lipid levels in hypertensive patients. J Cardiovasc Pharmacol 1984;6:S841-S846.

Kelton JG: Impaired reticuloendothelial function in patients treated with methyldopa. N Engl J Med 1985;313:596-600.

Korner PI, Head GA, Bobik A, Badoer E, Aberdeen JA: Central and peripheral autonomic mechanisms involved in the circulatory actions of methyldopa. Hypertension 1984;6(Suppl II):II-63-II-70.

Schaller M-D, Nussberger J, Waeber B, Porchet M, Brunner HR: Transdermal clonidine therapy in hypertensive patients. JAMA 1985;253:233-5.

Notes

#17 Adrenergic Inhibitors: Alpha-blockers

Currently, one drug in this class is available—prazosin (Minipress). More will probably be introduced in the near future, including Indoramin, Terazosin and Doxazosin.

Mode of Action

Prazosin has a much higher affinity for the post-synaptic alpha$_1$-receptors located on the vascular smooth muscle cells than on the pre-synaptic alpha$_2$-receptors located on the neuronal membrane. The selective uptake by the α_1-receptors blocks the uptake of catecholamines by the smooth muscle cells thereby blunting vasoconstriction and inducing peripheral vasodilation. The drug was originally thought to be a direct vasodilator but its vasodilatory action comes about via α_1-blockade (Figure 6).

The failure of prazosin to block the α_2-receptors on the neuron leaves them open to the effects of catecholamines present within the synaptic cleft. Thereby the release of additional norepinephrine (NE) from the neuronal storage granules is inhibited. Those non-selective alpha-blockers, phentolamine (Regitine) and phenoxybenzamine (Dibenzyline), which also block the neuronal α_2-receptors, remove the inhibitory effect upon NE release so more NE enters the circulation, blunting the antihypertensive effect and causing tachycardia. The latter drugs are only useful for therapy of pheochromocytoma.

Dosage

The initial dose of the drug may lower the blood pressure excessively, particularly in those already taking a diuretic. First-dose hypotension can be obviated by:

- Stopping the diuretic for 2 days before
- Giving only 1 mg of the drug
- Warning the patient about the possibility of postural symptoms

Some suggest taking the first dose at bedtime. To preclude trouble if the patient arises from bed during the night, the first dose may be taken on a day when the patient can lie around and better manage postural symptoms. In fact, the problem is very infrequent.

Dosage should be continued with 1 mg twice a day and can be raised to 10 mg twice a day.

Side Effects

Beyond the very rare first-dose hypotension, some patients continue to experience dizziness and a few others GI distress. The drug rarely causes CNS side effects such as sedation or dry mouth.

Lipid Effects

Beta-blockers often raise serum triglycerides and lower HDL-cholesterol levels (see Section 19). Alpha-blockers appear to do the opposite:

- Total cholesterol and triglyceride levels are lowered
- HDL-cholesterol is raised in many patients

Thus prazosin shares a lipid-protective effect with guanabenz although the manner by which they act is probably different.

Prazosin and other selective alpha$_1$-receptor blockers which may become available are particularly useful in young patients whose wish to remain physically active may preclude the use of beta-blockers which reduce exercise capacity by lowering cardiac output. This class of drugs provides good antihypertensive effects without worsening lipids or lowering potassium, as do diuretics.

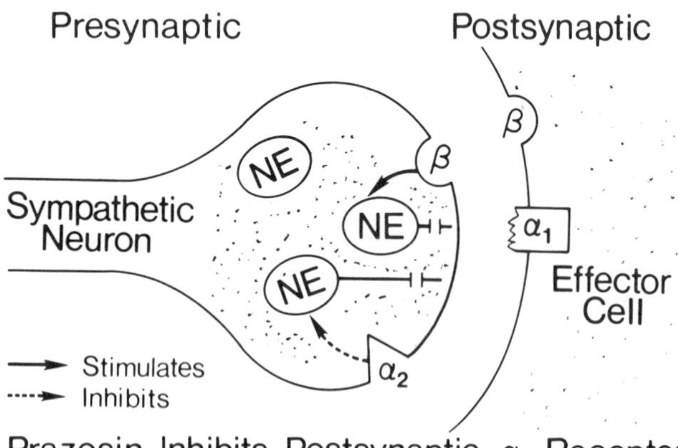

Prazosin Inhibits Postsynaptic α_1 Receptor But Not Presynaptic α_2 Receptor

FIGURE 6. A schematic representation of a neuron and a vascular smooth muscle cell, showing how prazosin preferentially blocks the α_1-receptor and leaves the presynaptic alpha$_2$-receptor unblocked. (From Kaplan NM. *Clinical Hypertension. 4th ed.* Baltimore: Williams & Wilkins, 1986).

References:

Leren P: Effect of alpha- and beta-blocker therapy on blood lipids: European experience. Am J Med 1984;76: (Suppl 2A):67-71.

Sacks FM, Dzau VJ: Adrenergic effects on plasma lipoprotein metabolism. Am J Med 1986;80 (suppl 2A):71-81.

Stanaszek WF, Kellerman D, Brogden RN, Romankiewicz JA: Prazosin update: a review of its pharmacological properties and therapeutic use in hypertension. Drugs 1983;25:339-84.

Van Zwieten PA, Timmermans PBMWM, Van Brummelen P: Role of alpha adrenoceptors in hypertension and in antihypertensive drug treatment. Am J Med 1984;77:17-25.

Velasco M, Silva H, Feldstein E, et al.: Effects of prazosin and alphamethyldopa on blood lipids and lipoproteins in hypertensive patients. Eur J Clin Pharmacol 1985;28:513-6.

Walker RG, Whitworth JA, Saines D, Kincaid-Smith P: Prazosin: long-term treatment of moderate and severe hypertension and lack of “tolerance”. Med J Aust 1981;2:146-7.

#18 Adrenergic Inhibitors: Beta-Blockers, Part I

This group of drugs has rapidly become the second most widely used after diuretics. They provide numerous benefits but the adverse effects on lipids need to be considered. Those which have partial agonist (or intrinsic sympathomimetic) activity (ISA) may provide all of the benefits with fewer of the adverse effects (Table 5).

Mode of Action

Those with no ISA lower the blood pressure by:

- Reducing cardiac output
- Inhibiting the release of renin
- Reducing norepinephrine release from neurons
- Decreasing central vasomotor activity (Figure 7).

In the peripheral vessels, beta-blockade inhibits vasodilation so that unopposed alpha-mediated vasoconstriction causes vascular resistance to increase. This limits the antihypertensive effect and is responsible for the side effect of cold extremities.

Those with ISA lower the blood pressure without reducing cardiac output and may decrease peripheral resistance by causing some sympathetic stimulation while blocking endogenous catechol effects. They cause less bradycardia and cold extremities.

Differences Between Beta-Blockers

Beyond different degrees of ISA, beta-blockers differ in lipid solubility and relative selectivity in blocking β_1-receptors in the heart versus β_2-receptors elsewhere.

Lipid Solubility

Propranolol, metoprolol and timolol are very lipid soluble, pindolol and acebutolol have intermediate lipid solubility, whereas atenolol and nadolol are much less lipid soluble. The more lipid soluble, the more of the drug that is taken up and metabolized on the first pass through the liver and the more of the drug that enters the brain. The greater hepatic uptake results in inactivation of the first few doses, until uptake is saturated. A small I.V. dose may produce much greater effects than a larger oral dose. Lipid-soluble agents generally have shorter duration of action because of more rapid hepatic inactivation. However, in the relatively large doses used to treat hypertension, most beta-blockers will provide 24 hour antihypertensive effects with one dose a day.

The lipid insoluble (or water soluble) agents remain unmetabolized in the blood and are slowly excreted through the kidneys; therefore, the duration of action is longer. Less enters the brain and they seem to have fewer CNS side effects.

Cardioselectivity

Acebutolol, atenolol and metoprolol are more active on cardiac β_1-receptors than on β_2-receptors. This selectivity can be shown with acute administration of single doses. These agents cause less decrease in peripheral blood flow or pulmonary air movement than non-cardioselective agents. However, none are truly cardioselective and most differences disappear with chronic use of larger doses.

Clinical Effectiveness

The antihypertensive effectiveness of the various beta-blockers in equivalent doses is similar.

When used alone, beta-blockers appear to be more effective in patients who are younger and white and less effective in elderly and blacks. This difference may reflect lower plasma renin levels in elderly and black patients.

Beta-blockers may be particularly useful in patients with:

- Hypertension associated with tachycardia and high cardiac output
- Hypertension accompanied by:
  - Angina
  - Migraine
  - Glaucoma
  - Other coincidental diseases which are responsive to beta-blockade

Beta-blockers have been shown to reduce recurrent myocardial infarction and sudden death among patients who recently experienced an acute MI. However they were not found to reduce the incidence of initial myocardial infarction in a large trial performed in Europe, the International Prospective Primary Prevention Study in Hypertension, where half of the hypertensives were given a β-blocker (Oxprenolol) and the other half were treated with various other drugs.

TABLE 5
PROPERTIES OF BETA-BLOCKERS

Generic Name	Trade Name	Cardio-Selectivity	Intrinsic Sympatho-mimetic Activity	Lipid Solubility
Acebutolol	Sectral	+	+	+
Alprenolol	Aptin	−	+	+ + +
Atenolol	Tenormin	+	−	−
Metoprolol	Lopressor	+	−	+ + +
Nadolol	Corgard	−	−	−
Oxprenolol	Trasicor	−	+	+ + +
Pindolol	Visken	−	+ +	+ +
Propranolol	Inderal	−	−	+ + +
Sotalol	Sotacor	−	−	+
Timolol	Blocarden	−	−	+ +

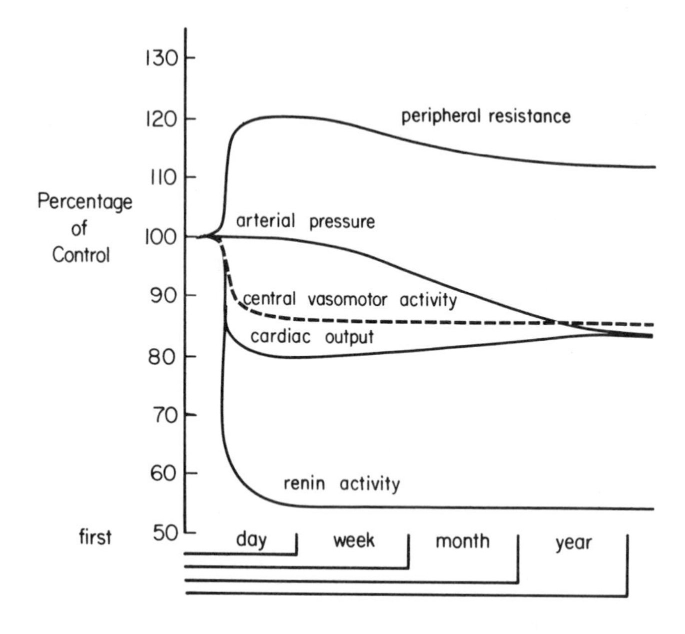

FIGURE 7. Schematic representation of the multiple actions of β-blocker therapy over variable periods of time. The solid lines have been measured; the dotted line of central vasomotor activity has not been measured. (Adapted from Birkenhager WH, et al. Therapeutic effects of β-adrenoceptor blocking agents in hypertension. In Frick P, et al. *Advances in Internal Medicine and Pediatrics, No. 39.* Berlin: Springer-Verlag, 1977:117-134.)

References:

IPPPSH Collaborative Group: Cardiovascular risk and risk factors in a randomized trial of treatment based on the beta-blocker oxprenolol: the International Prospective Primary Prevention Study in Hypertension (IPPPSH). J Hypertension 1985;3:379-92.

Leenen FHH, Boer P, Dorhout Mees EJ: Antihypertensive effect and degree of β-adrenoceptor blockade after short-term and semi-chronic propranolol therapy. Br J Clin Pharmac 1984;17:745-52.

Man in't Veld AJ, Schalekamp MADH: How intrinsic sympathomimetic activity modulates the haemodynamic responses to β-adrenoceptor antagonists; a clue to the nature of their antihypertensive mechanism. Br J Clin Pharmacol 1982;13:245S-7S.

Singh BN, Thoden WR, Ward A: Acebutolol: a review of its pharmacological properties and therapeutic efficacy in hypertension, angina pectoris and arrhythmia. Drugs 1985;29:531-69.

van Baak MA, Struyker Boudier HAJ, Smits JFM: Antihypertensive mechanisms of beta-adrenoceptor blockade: a review. Clin Exper Hypertension 1985;A7:1-72.

van der Veur E, ten Berge BS, Donker AJM, May JF, Schuurman FH, Wesseling H: Comparison of atenolol 50 mg and 100 mg as initial treatment in uncomplicated mild to moderate hypertension. Eur J Clin Pharmacol 1985;28:351-2.

#19 Adrenergic Inhibitors: Beta-Blockers, Part II

Beta-blockers may be associated with various side effects. Most are predictable in view of their pharmacological action. Some side effects are more common in those which are non-cardioselective or lipid soluble or which lack intrinsic sympathomimetic activity (ISA).

Cardiac

Those with no or little ISA induce bradycardia which may be asymptomatic and should be disregarded. Those who monitor the degree of physical activity by heart rate should be made aware that maximal heart rate will be approximately 20% lower. The state of physical conditioning can be achieved in the presence of beta-blockade, but reduced exercise ability and easier fatigue are often noted, less so with ISA beta-blockers.

Beta-blockers tend to slow the rate of A-V conduction and may worsen the degree of heart block.

The decrease in cardiac output with non-ISA beta-blockers may induce various side effects, sometimes referred to as "betacardia." A few patients, near decompensation already, may be pushed into congestive heart failure when using a β-blocker.

Pulmonary

Bronchospasm may result if patients are in need of β-agonist effects to maintain patent airways. Cardioselective β-blockers may decrease air movement; however if beta-agonist bronchodilators are required, they will be more effective in the presence of a more cardioselective β-blocker.

Metabolic

Diabetics who take insulin and are prone to hypoglycemia should be given β-blockers with great caution. The response to hypoglycemia largely depends upon catecholamine stimulation of glucose synthesis and release, particularly in insulin-dependent diabetics who are also unable to secrete glucagon. Insulin-induced hypoglycemia may be longer in duration and more severe in the presence of a β-blocker. The β-blockers mask the usual symptoms of hypoglycemia such as tremor, tachycardia and hunger, but not sweating. Diabetics given β-blockers should be aware of the significance of sweating as a warning signal.

Hypertriglyceridemia and a concomitant fall in HDL-cholesterol are common with β-blockers, though less marked or not at all with those having high degrees of ISA. Serum triglyceride levels rise an average of 30% with most β-blockers (Figure 8). These lipid abnormalities may be responsible for the failure of β-blocker therapy to reduce the incidence of coronary heart disease in controlled therapeutic trials.

Central

Fatigue is common. It may be related to the decreased cardiac output seen with non-ISA β-blockers or to central effects. Bad dreams, even hallucinations, may be noted. Depression has been increasingly recognized with the use of propranolol. These effects are less common with the lipid-insoluble agents and those with ISA.

Renal

A 10 to 20% fall in renal blood flow and glomerular filtration rate has been noted with most β-blockers, though not with nadolol. The effect may reflect renal vasoconstriction.

Fluid retention has been noted in a small number of low-renin hypertensives given propranolol.

An Overview of Beta-Blocker Therapy

In the past 10 years, β-blockers have been increasingly used as first or second drug in the treatment of hypertension. They are effective and usually well tolerated. However, they may cause fatigue and loss of exercise ability that many patients may not relate to the drug. Of more concern are the lipid abnormalities seen with those which lack ISA.

These drugs protect against recurrent MIs but have not been shown to protect against the first heart attack, with the possible exception of their use among men who do not smoke. The multiple side effects preclude their use in as many as 25% of patients. If a β-blocker is chosen, one with intrinsic sympathomimetic activity (ISA) would seem to be the best choice since it will probably cause fewer side effects which are clinically obvious and biochemically important.

References:

Avorn J, Everitt DE, Weiss S: Increased antidepressant use in patients prescribed β-blockers. JAMA 1986;255:357-60.

Bauer JH: Adrenergic blocking agents and the kidney. J Clin Hypertens 1985;3:199-221.

Dornhorst A, Powell SH, Pensky J: Aggravation by propranolol of hyperglycaemic effect of hydrochlorothiazide in type II diabetics without alteration of insulin secretion. Lancet 1985;1:123-6.

Epstein M, Oster JR: Beta blockers and renal function: a reappraisal. J Clin Hypertens 1985;1:85-99.

Gordon NF, van Rensburg JP, Russell HMS, et al.: Effect of $beta_1$ selective adrenoceptor blockade on physiological response to exercise. Br Heart J 1985;54:96-9.

Weidmann P, Uehlinger DE, Gerber A: Antihypertensive treatment and serum lipoproteins (Editorial Review). J Hypertension 1985;3:297-306.

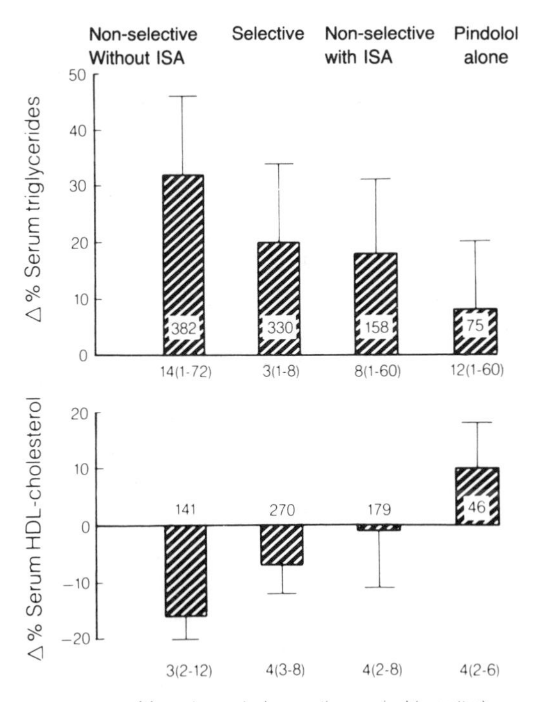

FIGURE 8. Mean percentage responses of serum triglycerides and HDL-cholesterol to monotherapy with different types of beta-blockers (mean ± s.d.). ISA - intrinsic sympathomimetic activity. Numbers in columns denote the total numbers of reported cases used for analysis (From Weidman P et al. J. Hypertension 1985;3:297).

#20 Adrenergic Inhibitors: Combined Alpha- and Beta-Blockers

Currently, only one drug, labetalol (Normodyne, Trandate) is available which has both alpha- and beta-blocking effects within the same structure. It is available for both oral and intravenous use.

Mode of Action

In smaller doses, the drug has three times more β-blocking effect than alpha-blocking action. A maximal degree of alpha-blockade occurs with increasing doses, whereas the beta-blocking effects continue so that the ratio increases to 6 to 1 or higher.

The beta-blocking actions are similar to that seen with propranolol, which is non-cardioselective and lipid soluble. The alpha-blocking effect is similar to those seen with prazosin, inducing peripheral vasodilation. As a result of the combination of effects, blood pressure falls mainly from a decrease in peripheral resistance with little effect on heart rate or cardiac output. Little change is noted in renin or catechol levels and renal function is not altered.

When taken by mouth, its lipid solubility results in extensive first pass hepatic metabolism so that only about 25% is bioavailable. The duration of action is 8 to 12 hours.

When given intravenously, the anti-hypertensive effect is rapid and may be profound, with a propensity to postural hypotension if the patients stands.

Dosage

By mouth, 200 mg twice a day is usually an adequate starting dose with a maximum of 2400 mg/day. By vein, the drug may be given initially in a 20 mg dose by slow injection, with repeated 20 to 80 mg doses at 10 minute intervals. The maximal effect of each dose is usually seen within 10 minutes and the duration of action is up to 6 hours. The drug may also be given by slow continuous infusion at an initial rate of 2 mg per minute, with 50 to 200 mg usually required for an adequate response.

Side Effects

Some side effects are related to alpha-blockade:

- Postural dizziness
- Scalp tingling
- Nasal stuffiness

Other side effects are related to beta-blockade:

- Fatigue
- Vivid dreams
- Bronchospasm
- Cold extremities
- Claudication

In addition, the drug may cause GI distress with:

- Nausea
- Vomiting
- Pain
- Diarrhea
- Constipation

Clinical Use

Orally, this drug should be used primarily for treatment of moderate and severe degrees of hypertension. Intravenously, it should be useful in those who have a need for rapid, though not instantaneous, reduction of markedly elevated blood pressure. Those who do not require nitroprusside but who need parenteral therapy can be given labetalol rather than diazoxide or hydralazine. This may be an advantage in being able to quickly switch the patient to chronic oral therapy with the same drug.

References:

Feit A, Holtzman R, Cohen M, El-Sherif N: Effect of labetalol on exercise tolerance and double product in mild to moderate essential hypertension. Am J Med 1985;78:937-41.

Lebel M, Langlois S, Belleau LJ, Grose JH: Labetalol infusion in hypertensive emergencies. Clin Pharmacol Ther 1985;37:615-8.

Louis WJ, McNeil JJ, Drummer OH: Pharmacology of combined α-β-blockade. Drugs 1984;28(Suppl 2):16-34.

Lund-Johansen P: Pharmacology of combined α-β-blockade II: haemodynamic effects of labetalol. Drugs 28(Suppl 2):35-50.

Prichard BNC: Combined α- and β-receptor inhibition in the treatment of hypertension. Drugs 1984;28 (Suppl 2):51-68.

Notes

#21 Vasodilators: Direct-Acting

Two drugs in this group, hydralazine and minoxidil, directly dilate arterioles. Others whose effects are similar but whose modes of action are different include the converting enzyme inhibitors and the calcium antagonists (see Sections 22 and 23 and Table 6).

The use of direct-acting vasodilators has been made practical by combining them with diuretics and adrenergic inhibitors (Figure 9). Serapes is such a combination of small amounts of hydralazine with hydrochlorothiazide and reserpine. Serapes has been available for a long time and remains useful for patients with mild-moderate hypertension. During the last 10 years, larger doses of hydralazine and minoxidil have been used as part of triple therapy to treat severe degrees of hypertension.

These drugs alone induce significant dilation of resistance arterioles with a fall in peripheral resistance. The resultant fall in blood pressure activates baroreceptors which set off sympathetic reflexes causing:

- Stimulation of the heart
- Constriction of veins
- Release of both renin and catecholamines

The fall in blood pressure also leads to renal retention of sodium, expanding fluid volume.

Various side effects, e.g. tachycardia, flushing, headaches and a loss of antihypertensive efficacy are seen as a result of all of these compensatory reactions to the vasodilator-induced fall in blood pressure (Figure 9). With the concomitant use of an adrenergic inhibitor and a diuretic, the various compensatory reactions are inhibited and the blood pressure falls even more, thus reducing side effects. A beta-blocker may be used as the adrenergic inhibitor; however others such as clonidine or guanabenz may also be used. A thiazide is usually chosen as the diuretic but furosemide may be needed in those who have a marked response to minoxidil, particularly if they start with some degree of renal insufficiency.

Clinical Use

Hydralazine is often chosen as the third drug for those not responding adequately to a diuretic and an adrenergic inhibitor. The initial dose is usually 25 mg twice a day and may be increased to 200 mg twice a day although total daily doses beyond 200 mg are associated with an increasing likelihood of a lupus-like reaction.

Minoxidil is often used for patients with severe hypertension, particularly when renal insufficiency is present. It can be given once a day with total dosage from 5 to 60 mg. Its use is complicated by a marked tendency for:

- Fluid retention — requiring use of potent diuretics
- Hirsutism — precluding use of the drug in many women unwilling to have hair on their faces and elsewhere

Men are rarely concerned and the drug is being investigated for use as a topical treatment to regrow hair on bald heads.

Side Effects

Most side effects are directly attributable to the activation of compensatory mechanisms to direct vasodilation, including tachycardia, flushing and headache. However, hydralazine also can cause a lupus-like reaction with fever, rash and arthralgias but rarely renal or CNS involvement. The reaction is usually benign and disappears when the drug is stopped. Perry et al found that patients who have a reaction have no residual damage and a 10 to 15 year longer survival rate than similar patients who have not had a reaction.

The tendency for fluid retention and hirsutism with minoxidil reflects its marked vasodilation of renal and skin arterioles.

An Overview

These drugs are effective and generally well tolerated. However their use will probably recede in the face of equally effective CEIs and calcium antagonists which tend to cause fewer side effects.

TABLE 6
CHARACTERISTICS OF VASODILATORS

Drug	Trade Name	Dose Range (mg/day)	Side Effects
Direct Vasodilators			
Hydralazine	Apresoline	50-400	Headaches, tachycardia (if used alone), lupus-like syndrome
Minoxidil	Loniten	5-100	Headaches, fluid retention, hirsutism
Calcium Entry Blockers			
Nifepidine	Procardia	20-120	Flush, headache, local ankle edema
Verapamil	Isoptin, Calan	240-480	Constipation, headache, conduction defects
Diltiazem	Cardizem	120-240	Nausea, headache, conduction defects
Converting-Enzyme Inhibitors			
Captopril	Capoten	25-150	Rash, loss of taste Rare: leukopenia, proteinuria
Enalapril	Vasotec	5-20	All of above likely less common Rare: Angioneurotic edema

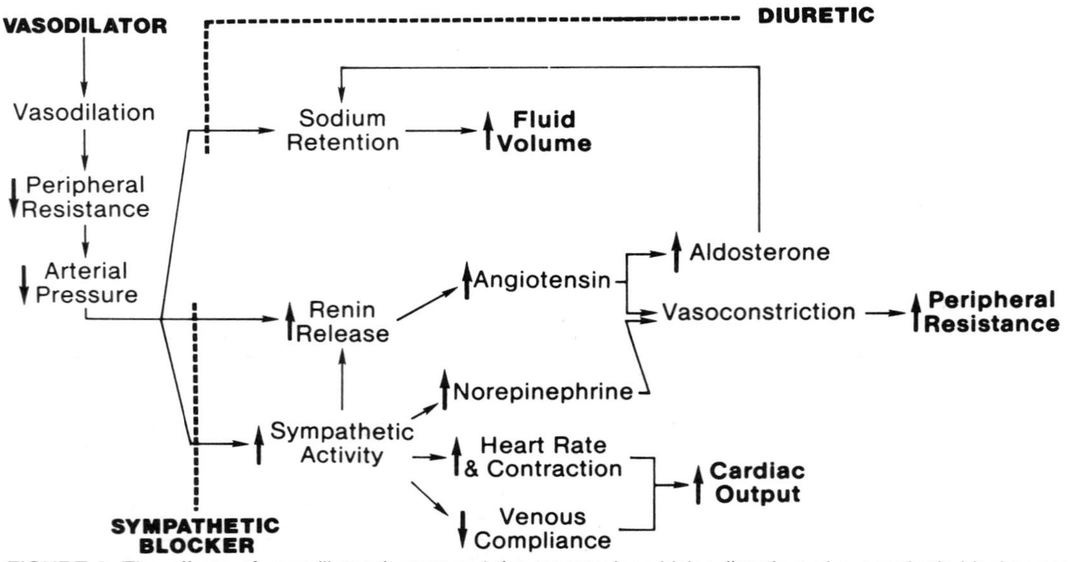

FIGURE 9. The effects of vasodilator therapy and the manner by which a diuretic and sympathetic blocker can overcome the undesirable secondary effects. (Adapted from Koch-Weser J. Arch Intern Med 1974;133:1017. Copyright 1974, American Medical Association.)

References:

Eggertsen R, Hansson L: Vasodilators in hypertension - a review with special emphasis on the combined use of vasodilators and beta-adrenoceptor blockers. Int J Clin Pharmacol Ther Toxicol 1985;23:411-23.

Mansilla-Tinoco R, Harland SJ, Ryan PJ, et al.: Hydralazine, antinuclear antibodies, and the lupus syndrome. Br Med J 1982;284:936-9.

Oh MS, Uribarri J, Alveranga D, Bazilinski N, Lazar I, Carroll HJ: Minoxidil in a once-a-day step-3 antihypertensive program. J Clin Hypertens 1985;1:23-9.

Perry HM Jr, Camel GH, Carmody SE, Ahmed KS, Perry EF: Survival in hydralazine-treated hypertensive patients with and without late toxicity. J Chron Dis 1977;30:519-28.

Silas JH, Ramsay LE, Freestone S: Hydralazine once daily in hypertension. Br Med J 1982;284:1602-4.

Taverner D, Bing RF, Heagerty A, et al.: Improvement of renal function during long-term treatment of severe hypertension with minoxidil. Quart J Med 1983;206:280-7.

#22 Vasodilators: Calcium Antagonists

This group of drugs includes the following:

- Diltiazem (Cardizem)
- Nifedipine (Procardia)
- Verapamil (Calan, Isoptin)

Each has a different chemical structure, site of action, and pharmacological properties. Even though not approved by the FDA for use in treatment of hypertension, they have been increasingly used for that purpose. A number of other calcium antagonists, most of which are dihydropyridines similar to nifedipine, are under investigation.

Mode of Action

Though they each work in a different manner, all three lower the blood pressure by reducing calcium entry into vascular smooth muscle cells. Some prefer the name "calcium channel" or "entry blockers" to "calcium antagonists." Regardless of the differences in their mode of action, all cause a decrease in free intracellular calcium which reduces vascular tone and contractility. Peripheral resistance and blood pressure fall.

Diltiazem and verapamil also act within the S-A and A-V nodes, making them useful for the treatment of certain arrhythmias but adding to their interaction with beta-blockers to induce serious A-V conduction block. Nifedipine has no effect upon sinus or A-V nodal conduction. This is an advantage in reducing β-blocker interactions and a disadvantage in allowing for some reflex tachycardia.

Clinical Use

Currently, all three are available in the U.S. in fairly short acting formulations. Three doses per day must be used for a sustained 24 hour anti-hypertensive effect. Longer lasting preparations are currently available elsewhere and will probably be in the U.S in the near future. These drugs have been found by some to work better in older patients than in younger patients and particularly well in blacks.

Nifedipine and diltiazem work more quickly than verapamil. Considerable experience with nifedipine, given either sublingually or swallowed, has shown that it lowers blood pressure markedly within 20 minutes.

Side Effects

The nature and severity of side effects differ considerably among the three drugs, reflecting different effects at various sites such as peripheral vasodilation (nifedipine > veramapil > diltiazem) and A-V conduction (verapamil > diltiazem, nifedipine none at all). The most common side effects with each include:

- Diltiazem:
  - Nausea
  - Ankle edema
  - Headache
  - Rash
- Nifedipine:
  - Flushing
  - Headache
  - Postural dizziness
  - Nausea
  - Ankle edema

- Verapamil:
  - Constipation
  - Postural dizziness
  - Headache
  - Nausea

The edema is not generalized and is localized to the ankles or legs, likely secondary to vasodilation. It may be so cosmetically bothersome as to preclude the use of these drugs, particularly nifedipine.

Verapamil is most likely to cause myocardial depression, excessive bradycardia or AV nodal dysfunction and should rarely be used with beta-blockers.

Although the secretion of most hormones is dependent upon local release of calcium, hormonal secretions are affected very little by these drugs and they may be safely used in diabetics.

An Overview

Calcium antagonists are effective antihypertensives. They will probably be widely used when available as once or twice a day preparations, particularly if they produce smoother antihypertensive action. As of now, the need to give them three times a day has limited their use mainly to those with more severe hypertension who are resistant or bothered by other drugs. The potential to protect against both cardiac and vascular damage as shown experimentally and the ability to reduce the blood pressure particularly well in elderly patients as shown in a few clinical trials, suggest that calcium antagonists may become very popular antihypertensive agents.

References:

Brouwer RML, Follath F, Buhler FR: Review of the cardiovascular adversity of the calcium antagonist beta-blocker combination: implications for antihypertensive therapy. J Cardiovasc Pharmacol 1985;7(Suppl 4):S38-S44.

Buhler FR, Bolli P, Erne P, et al.: Position of calcium antagonists in antihypertensive therapy. J Cardiovasc Pharmacol 1985;7(Suppl 4):S21-S27.

Chaffman M, Brogden RN: Diltiazem: a review of its pharmacological properties and therapeutic efficacy. Drugs 1985;29:387-454.

Halperin AK, Cubeddu LX: The role of calcium channel blockers in the treatment of hypertension. Am Heart J 1986;111:347-52.

Henry PD: Atherosclerosis, calcium, and calcium antagonists. Circulation 1985;72:456-9.

M'Buyamba-Kabangu JR, Lepira B, Fagard R, et al.: Relative potency of a beta-blocking and a calcium entry blocking agent as antihypertensive drugs in black patients. Eur J Clin Pharmacol 1986;29:523-7.

Robinson BF: Calcium-entry blocking agents in the treatment of systemic hypertension. Am J Cardiol 1985;55:102B-106B.

Sorkin EM, Clissold SP, Brogden RN: Nifedipine: a review of its pharmacodynamic and pharmacokinetic properties, and therapeutic efficacy, in ischaemic heart disease, hypertension and related cardiovascular disorders. Drugs 1985;30:182-274.

van Zwieten PA, Timmermans PBMWM: Pharmacological basis of the antihypertensive action of calcium entry blockers. J Cardiovasc Pharmacol 1985;7(Suppl 4):S11-S17.

#23 Vasodilators: Converting Enzyme Inhibitors

Only captopril has been previously available, but enalapril has recently been released and a large number are under clinical investigation. As a group, they provide excellent antihypertensive action with few bothersome side effects. However, initial experiences with captopril reported a high frequency of serious side effects. The drug was originally introduced for therapy of resistant hypertension only. When used in such patients, who often required large doses of drugs and had significant pre-existing renal damage, side effects were common and often serious. The frequency and severity of side effects have fallen progressively as the drug has been given in smaller doses to patients with milder hypertension and good renal function. Captopril is now approved for use for all degrees of hypertension as is enalapril.

Mode of Action (Figure 10)

The conversion of the inactive prohormone angiotensin I to the potent vasoconstrictor angiotensin II (A-II) is accomplished by an angiotensin converting enzyme (ACE) available throughout the body. By ingenious molecular manipulation, biochemists engineered a drug which competitively inhibited the converting enzyme by attaching to its binding sites on the angiotensin I structure. The CEI completely inhibits the synthesis of angiotensin II and all of the effects of the hormone are countered. A-II-mediated vasoconstriction is overcome, so the blood pressure falls. A-II-mediated synthesis of aldosterone is inhibited, thereby sodium retention and potassium wastage are reduced.

ACE is the same enzyme which inactivates

the vasodepressor hormone bradykinin. Inhibition of this inactivation by CEI may allow the vasodepressor effect to persist so this effect may be involved in the antihypertensive action of the drug. In addition, captopril (but not enalapril) appears to directly stimulate the synthesis of vasodilatory prostaglandins in renal and vascular endothelium.

Peripheral resistance and the blood pressure fall as a result of these effects. Cardiac output does not increase, possibly because of inhibition of the expected baroreceptor-mediated reflex increase in sympathetic activity as a result of the absence of angiotensin II. Despite marked falls in blood pressure, heart rate rarely rises.

The ability to reduce systemic vascular resistance without cardiac stimulation makes CEIs particularly useful as unloading agents in the treatment of severe congestive heart failure.

Clinical Use

Increasingly, smaller doses of captopril (12 1/2 to 25 mg twice to three times a day) are being used to treat milder degrees of hypertension. Small doses should be used as initial therapy in those suspected of high renin-angiotensin forms of hypertension since they may experience a precipitous first-dose hypotension when the support of the blood pressure by A-II is acutely removed. In particular, patients with renovascular hypertension, wherein high levels of A-II have served to maintain renal blood flow past the stenoses, may experience a marked fall in blood pressure and loss of renal function with CEI therapy. Patients with unilateral renovascular hypertension tend to respond well to the drug and it is the usual choice for medical therapy.

Side Effects

Side effects may be related to:

- Pharmacological effect of the drugs
  - Hypotension
  - Loss of renal function
- Related to the sulfhydryl group contained within captopril but not in enalapril
  - Rash
  - Loss of taste
  - Glomerulopathy with proteinuria
  - Leukopenia

The latter symptoms seem to be less common with enalapril but the difference may reflect the wider exposure of patients to high doses of captopril.

Overview

These agents probably will become widely used in the treatment of milder degrees of hypertension as well as the more severe, resistant forms. They work particularly well in those with higher renin levels including those on diuretics. Research in animals shows the agents may protect against renal damage better than other drugs that lower the blood pressure as well. Research in patients with high-normal renin levels suggest that they may correct an underlying fault of tissue responsiveness to A-II. The outlook seems particularly promising. The potential to cause serious side effects, however, should not be forgotten.

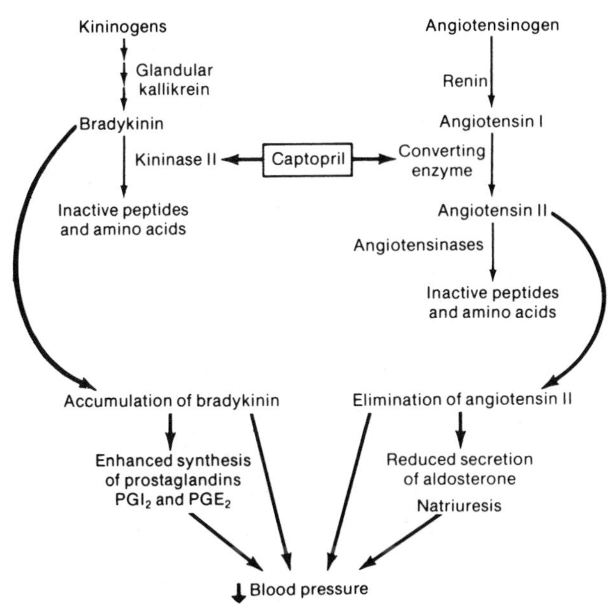

FIGURE 10. The mechanisms by which captopril and other converting enzyme inhibitors may lower the blood pressure. (From Kaplan NM, *Clinical Hypertension. 4th ed.* Baltimore: Williams & Wilkins, 1986.)

References:

Brunner HR, Nussberger J, Waeber B: Effects of angiotensin converting enzyme inhibition: a clinical point of view. J Cardiovasc Pharmacol 1985;7(Suppl 4):S73-S81.

Kromer EP, Riegger GAJ, Liebau G, Kochsiek K: Effectiveness of converting enzyme inhibition (enalapril) for mild congestive heart failure. Am J Cardiol 1986;57:549-62.

Laragh JH: When is it useful to inhibit the renin-angiotensin system for treating hypertension? J Cardiovasc Pharmacol 1985;7(Suppl 4):S86-S91.

Williams GH, Hollenberg NK: Are non-modulating patients with essential hypertension a distinct subgroup? Am J Med 1985;79(Suppl 3C):3-9.

#24 Step-Care or Multiple Choice and Substitution

Most American practitioners have used the Step-Care approach to therapy: start with one drug and add a second, a third and a fourth in sequence if the response is inadequate. For most, the first step has been a thiazide diuretic and this group of drugs has become the most widely prescribed in the U.S. Elsewhere, diuretics are less commonly chosen as first drug.

The diuretic-first, step-care approach was recommended in the 1977 and 1980 reports of the U.S. Joint National Committee (JNC), a group of hypertension experts appointed by the head of the National Heart, Lung and Blood Institute to formulate guidelines for the detection, evaluation and treatment of hypertension. The 1984 report of the Third JNC broadened the choice of first drug to either a diuretic or a beta-blocker, with less than full doses as the first step. If the full dose of diuretic or beta-blocker was inadequate, the addition of the other one was recommended as the next step. The Committee recommended that adrenergic inhibitors other than beta-blockers could be chosen for selected patients.

Additional Choices

Although this approach has worked well, there are now reasons to add additional choices and to discard the rigid step-care regimen widely used in the U.S. Choices other than diuretics or beta-blockers will be shown perhaps to provide better long-term protection against coronary disease because they do not adversely alter potassium as do diuretics or alter lipids as do diuretics and beta-blockers (see Sections 13 and 19).

A Substitution Approach

In addition to broadening the choice of first drug, consideration should be given to a different approach than the step-wise addition of a second drug if the first proves inadequate. Although it is true that all antihypertensive drugs approved for use have similar efficacy for the overall hypertensive population, there are differences in response to different drugs among certain groups of patients and between individual patients.

24.

For example, younger and white patients generally respond better to an adrenergic inhibitor or a converting enzyme inhibitor. Older and black patients respond better to a diuretic or a calcium antagonist. These differences may reflect differences in plasma renin activity or the differing contributions of various pathogenetic mechanisms.

Beyond these general differences, individual patients of the same type may respond variably to any one drug. What works well for one elderly black female may do very little for another. Rather than immediately adding another drug as second step, the wiser course may be to stop the first drug which has proved ineffectual and try another from another class of drugs. The number of drugs will be minimized and effectiveness will be maximized.

The step-care approach seems more appropriate for patients with significant hypertension, wherein the first drug provides a definite effect but not enough to bring the considerably elevated pressure to the goal of therapy. Although any given dose of antihypertensive agent will apparently be more effective the higher the initial blood pressure, it should be noted that most drugs have a limited efficacy. The addition of a second or third drug is indicated if a partial but definite effect has been achieved with the first drug.

80% of all hypertensives are in the mild category, i.e. DBP between 90 and 104 mm Hg. Half of these (40% of all hypertensive patients) have DBP between 90 and 95 mm Hg (Figure 1). For these, one drug may be enough to accomplish a 5 to 10 mm Hg fall in DBP. If the first drug does not accomplish the goal, another should be substituted rather than added.

References:

Buhler FR, Bolli P, Kiowski W, Erne P, Hulthan UL, Block LH: Renin profiling to select antihypertensive baseline drugs: renin inhibitors for high-renin and calcium entry blockers for low-renin patients. Am J Med 1984;77:36-42.

Gifford RW Jr: The role of diuretics in the treatment of hypertension. Am J Med 1984;77:102-6.

Laragh JH: Lessons from antihypertensive drug trials that employed "stepped care": the case for rationalized individualized treatment strategies based on renin system patterns. J Cardiovasc Pharmacol 1984;6:S1067-S1072.

Notes

#25 The Choice of First Drug

A large number of drugs can be chosen for initial therapy. The choice should be made carefully. If the patient responds well, the drug may be taken for many years, therefore inapparent biochemical and other side effects must be avoided. If the patient does not respond well or has significant side effects with the first drug, he may be dissuaded from returning for followup care.

The majority of patients have mild hypertension which should be adequately managed with one drug. In most of the therapeutic trials involving patients with DBP from 90 up to 109 mm Hg, 40 to 60% of patients had pressures brought to below 90 (and often had at least a 10 mm Hg absolute fall) with one drug. The choice of the first drug is therefore an important one.

Past Choices

A thiazide diuretic has been the usual first choice in the U.S. more than elsewhere. However, a number of concerns have risen about their use, particularly in the high doses often prescribed:

- In various therapeutic trials, wherein diuretics were the first and often only drug, protection against coronary disease has not been uniformly seen. In half of these trials, more coronary mortality, mostly due to sudden death, was seen among the treated patients (see Section 11)
- Diuretic-induced hypokalemia has sometimes been shown to invoke ventricular ectopic activity suggesting this as a mechanism for the increase in sudden deaths in the trials

- The 10 to 20 mg/dl rise in serum cholesterol seen with diuretics may counter the long-term protection against coronary disease provided by the lowered blood pressure

Present Choices

Partially as a result of these concerns, other drugs have been increasingly used, including beta-blockers, alpha-blockers and central agonists. These also may pose problems. Some believe diuretics in smaller doses remain the easiest and best initial therapy with proper surveillance and correction of the biochemical changes which may be induced. Combination with a potassium-sparing agent should make the diuretics even safer. The use of low dose thiazide plus triamterene in the European Trial in the Elderly did provide protection against coronary disease, unlike what was seen in some of the trials using high doses of diuretic without potassium-sparing agents.

However, many now use a beta-blocker, particuarly in younger patients who tend to be more responsive to them than the elderly. Awareness of the likelihood that the most widely used beta-blockers, such as propranolol, atenolol, and metoprolol, will raise serum triglycerides and lower HDL-cholesterol has raised concern about their use. Particularly among younger patients, the rather common complaints of fatigue and decrease in exercise ability and the lipid derangements, make them less attractive. Those beta-blockers with ISA, acebutolol and pindolol, may cause fewer side effects and should find increasing use as initial therapy.

Central agonists remain popular. Either clonidine or guanabenz provide all of the antihypertensive effect but none of the auto-immune inflammatory reactions seen with methyldopa. Guanabenz has been shown to lower serum cholesterol. However, sedation and dry mouth may make these difficult for some patients to take.

Alpha-blockers, with prazosin the only currently available member of this class, are an attractive choice. They act like a vasodilator: cardiac output is well maintained with no loss of exercise ability. They do not adversely alter lipids and, in many studies, prazosin monotherapy has been associated with lower total serum cholesterol and higher HDL-cholesterol levels. If used without a diuretic, first-dose and later postural hypotension is seldom a problem.

Future Choices

Along with these, CEIs and calcium antagonists will likely be widely used for initial therapy. Both act as vasodilators and neither reduce cardiac output nor appear to adversely alter blood lipids. With smaller doses, CEIs cause fewer bothersome or serious side effects and will likely be even more widely used now that a once a day CEI is available. Once a day calcium antagonists will probably also be available. Initial experiences suggest that calcium antagonists are more effective in older patients, thus particularly useful for treatment of the elderly.

References:

Amery A, Brixko P, Clement D, De Schaepdryver A, Fagard R, et al.: Mortality and morbidity results from the European Working Party on High Blood Pressure in the Elderly Trial. Lancet 1985;1:1349-54.

Freis ED: Choice for initial treatment. J Cardiovasc Pharmacol 1985;7:S112-S116.

Kaplan NM: Therapy of mild hypertension: an overview. Am J Cardiol 1984;53:2A-8A.

Krakoff LR: Antihypertensive treatment: cardiovascular risks and monotherapy. J Cardiovasc Pharmacol 1984;6:S833-S836.

Laragh JH: Modification of stepped care approach to antihypertensive therapy. Am J Med 1984;77:78-86.

#26 The Choice of Second Drug

Whatever agent other than a diuretic is chosen as first drug, a diuretic will often be chosen as second. The addition of a diuretic will increase the antihypertensive efficacy of other types of drugs. This reflects not only the expected antihypertensive effect derived from the action of the diuretic but also the ability of the diuretic to remove excess fluid that may have been retained by the kidneys of hypertensive patients when blood pressure is reduced. In addition to overcoming this "side effect" of non-diuretic therapy, the combination may blunt some of the side effects of the diuretic. If the initial choice has been either a beta-blocker or a CEI, the hypokalemia often induced by the diuretic may be prevented, presumably because these drugs block the diuretic-induced rises in renin-aldosterone. No information is available as to whether the prevention of potassium wastage will also prevent the hypercholesterolemic effect of diuretics.

Small Versus Large Doses

Before further consideration of the individual choices and combinations, a more general question needs attention: should maximal doses of the first drug be used before a second, or should smaller doses of two (or even more) drugs be used? Arguments can be made for either course.

In favor of maximal doses of the first are these: patients are more likely to take one medication and most medications come in single larger-dose tablets. If partial success is achieved with a smaller dose, more success is likely with a large dose. If the patient has had no problem with the initial dose, little trouble should be seen with increasing dosage.

In favor of smaller doses of two (or more drugs) are these: most antihypertensive drugs have a fairly flat dose-response curve. Most of the antihypertensive effect of hydrochlorothiazide is achieved with 25 mg a day and raising the dose to 50 or even 100 mg provides relatively little additional antihypertensive effect. Side effects are often dose-related. Fifty or 100 mg of HCT will cause increasingly more potassium wastage (Figure 3). Appropriate combinations of smaller doses of two antihypertensive agents, usually a diuretic plus another, are available and no more tablets or doses need to be taken.

There is no certain right answer. The step-care approach was predicated in part upon the concept that addition of second and third drugs in smaller doses was preferable to larger doses of single agents.

The Available Choices

Although diuretics will probably be added as second drug if a non-diuretic is the first, many patients will be given a diuretic as initial therapy. The choices of second drug include any of the adrenergic inhibitors, a CEI or a calcium antagonist. Few will tolerate effective doses of a direct vasodilator (hydralazine or minoxidil) in the absence of an adrenergic inhibitor to blunt the reflex sympathetic activity that usually accompanies the lowering of blood pressure by vasodilation. As noted in Sections 22 and 23, neither CEI nor calcium antagonists tend to activate baroreceptors as much as do the direct vasodilators, though they act as vasodilators. Baroreceptor reactivity tends to become blunted with age. Elderly patients may tolerate direct vasodilators when given alone or with a diuretic.

Two Drugs Without a Diuretic

If the initial drug is an adrenergic inhibitor, the second need not be a diuretic, particularly in patients with gout, diabetes, irritable hearts or other circumstances where the biochemical side effects of diuretics need to be avoided. The choice could be another adrenergic inhibitor that acts in a different manner or a vasodilator. There is no reason to add a second drug that works in the same manner as the first, such as clonidine plus methyldopa or two beta-blockers. But an alpha-blocker could be added to a beta-blocker or the patient switched to the combined alpha-beta blocker labetalol; or a beta-blocker could be added to a central agonist, and so on.

The addition of a vasodilator as second drug when the initial drug is an adrenergic inhibitor may be more logical. The one exception would be if prazosin is the first drug since its effect, though mediated by alpha-blockade, is as a vasodilator. Though more vasodilation may be achieved by adding another vasodilator that acts in a different manner, the better choice would likely be one from another class of drug.

References:

Joint National Committee on Detection, Evaluation and Treatment of High Blood Pressure: The 1984 Report of the Joint National Committee on Detection, Evaluation, and Treatment of High Blood Pressure: Arch Intern Med 1984;144:1045-57.

van Schaik BAM, Geyskes GC, Kettner N, Boer P, Dorhout Mees EJ: Comparison of enalapril and propranolol in essential hypertension. Eur J Clin Pharmacol 1986;29:511-16.

Weinberger MH: Blood pressure and metabolic responses to hydrochlorothiazide, captopril, and the combination in black and white mild-to-moderate hypertensive patients. J Cardiovasc Pharmacol 1985;7:S52-55.

#27 The Choice of Third Drug

Perhaps 10% of hypertensive patients will require more than two drugs to achieve adequate control of the blood pressure. The same arguments for and against adding three drugs in smaller doses rather than taking two drugs to their highest doses can be made, with the exception of being able to provide all three in one tablet. The only single tablet containing 3 drugs in the U.S. is Serapes. The dose of both reserpine and hydrochlorothiazide would be excessive with more than three tablets a day as would be required to provide adequate control of significantly high blood pressure.

The Logical Combinations

Most use one of each of the following major categories when triple therapy is needed:

- Diuretic
- Adrenergic inhibitor
- Vasodilator

In the recent past, hydralazine has been the most popular vasodilator, with minoxidil reserved for those with renal insufficiency. In the future, either a CEI or a calcium antagonist will likely be chosen instead. Prazosin may be used as the vasodilator component of triple therapy since it acts in that manner.

Which is Best

Which of these various combinations is best? There are no properly conducted clinical trials to provide the answer. One study, by McAreavey et al, compared 5 different drugs (hydralazine, labetalol, methyldopa, minoxidil and prazosin) and a placebo in 240 patients whose DBP remained above 95 mm Hg on a full dose of a diuretic and a beta-blocker. The six choices were allocated in a random manner, each to about 40 of the patients. Those given the combined alpha-beta blocker labetalol had their beta-blocker stopped and only men were given minoxidil. The protocol precluded any change in the dose of diuretic or beta-blocker, with the third drug added in progressively larger doses to a pre-determined maximum. Each patient was treated for six months and the effect on blood pressure, as well as the number of patients able to continue on each drug, were determined.

As seen in Figure 11, minoxidil was clearly the most effective drug. But the design of the trial, which precluded increases in diuretic therapy, caused all but ten of the minoxidil treated patients to stop the drug because of fluid retention. The other four drugs were equal in their anti-hypertensive effect, all superior to placebo. However, fewer than half given labetalol or methyldopa were able to continue them for 6 months. Three-fourths of those given either hydralazine or prazosin were able to complete the trial.

This trial is the only one of its kind and was begun before either CEIs or calcium antagonists were available. In view of the difficulty in doing such controlled studies, it is unlikely that more will be done. The choice of third drug will have to continue to be made on logical assumptions as to which is better.

The Need for More Diuretic

The results with minoxidil indicate the frequent need for additional diuretic, often potent loop diuretics, to overcome the marked renal fluid retention that may follow successful reduction of the blood pressure with the potent vasodilator. Similar, though less striking, fluid retention may accompany the use of other drugs. Doses of diuretic that may have seemed adequate initially may no longer be enough. Despite all of the prior warnings about excessive diuretic therapy, there may be a need to give more to patients whose response to other drugs seems to be inadequate or fading.

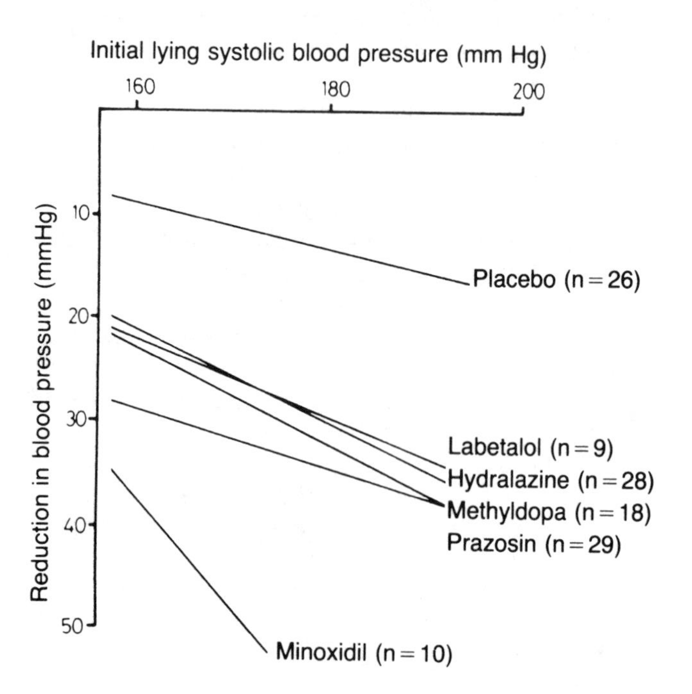

FIGURE 11. Regression lines relating reduction in blood pressure to initial lying systolic pressure for each drug group in randomized trial of placebo and 5 drugs in patients whose DBP remained > 95 on diuretic and beta-blocker. N in parentheses refers to number of patients in each group who were able to complete the study. (From McAreavery D, Ramsey LE, Lathem, et al. Br Med J 1984;288:106.)

References:

Guazzi MD, De Cesare N, Galli C, et al.: Calcium-channel blockade with nifedipine and angiotensin converting-enzyme inhibition with captopril in the therapy of patient with severe primary hypertension. Circulation 1984;70:279-84.

McAreavey D, Ramsey LE, Latham L, et al.: "Third drug" trial: comparative study of antihypertensive agents added to treatment when blood pressure remains uncontrolled by a beta blocker plus thiazide diuretic. Br Med J 1984;288:106-11.

#28 Step-Down Therapy And Drug Side Effects, With Emphasis on Impotence

STEP-DOWN THERAPY

Just as a minority of patients may be resistant to therapy, a large percentage of patients may be so sensitive as to be able to reduce the level of medication. In carefully controlled follow-up studies, about 15% of patients whose hypertension was well controlled on medications for 5 years have remained normotensive for up to 5 years after therapy was completely discontinued. In an on-going study of a group of such patients who were enrolled in the Hypertension Detection and Followup Program, the percentage whose pressures remain down is greater if they lose weight or reduce dietary sodium intake.

It is unknown why some patients who have not lost weight, reduced sodium intake, etc. are able to stop therapy, assuming they were truly hypertensive when therapy was started. The argument can be made that, since only 15% will remain normotensive off therapy, successful therapy should not be stopped, particularly because of the potential hazard of recurrence and progression of hypertension if the patient does not remain under observation. A larger group of patients whose pressures become normotensive on therapy may be able to reduce the level of therapy, i.e. step-down, rather than stop therapy altogether. This may occur because the patient is following one or more of the non-drug therapies described in Sections 9 and 10 or because the underlying mechanisms responsible for the development of hypertension have become quiescent or have been reversed by the lowering of pressure for some time. It may be that pressor mechanisms become more responsive to the actions of drugs. All who have been normotensive for a year or longer should attempt to reduce the dosage of medication. If more than one medication is being taken, only one should be reduced at a time. In one study, the dose of diuretic could be halved in most patients without a loss of blood pressure control but with a reduction in diuretic-induced hypokalemia.

IMPOTENCE

Of various side effects of therapy (Table 7), inability to gain and maintain an erection is perhaps the least well understood and managed. Most of the individual side effects are related to the mode of action of the various drugs. Loss of erectile potency may accompany the use of any antihypertensive agent. In the first 2 years of the MRC trial, impotence was noted in 10% of men on placebo, 13% on a beta-blocker, and 23% on a thiazide diuretic.

This surprisingly higher frequency with diuretic therapy may reflect the greater blood pressure lowering effect initially observed with diuretics in the MRC trial. Hypertensive men may have considerable atherosclerotic narrowing of the arteries bringing blood into the penis. Penile blood flow may diminish further if the head of pressure within this area of the circulation is reduced significantly by effective antihypertensive therapy more so than elsewhere. Since erection requires a 10-fold increase in blood flow, the occurence of impotence can be looked upon as a non-specific effect of successful lowering of the blood pressure.

Certain drugs, particularly central alpha agonists, may cause more impotence by interfering with neurogenic control of penile function. Impotence may be purely psychogenic, reflecting the concerns of middle-aged men who suddenly find themselves to have hypertension. But many become impotent because their pressures are brought down too much and too fast. In common with cerebral blood flow, too great and sudden a fall in blood pressure may cause tissue hypoperfusion. Therefore, the lowering of blood pressure should be gradual and gentle. If impotence appears with any one drug, the patients should discontinue use of the drug and be watched to see if potency returns. If it does, another type of drug should be used. The switch of therapy can be made if the pressure is so high as not to allow discontinuation of therapy, with encouragement that the switch may make a difference.

Loss of sexual desire or libido is rarely an organic problem caused by antihypertensive medications and is more likely psychogenic in origin. A drug such as spironolactone which can interfere with testosterone synthesis may cause loss of libido.

References:

Bancroft J, Wu FC: Erectile impotence. Br Med J 1985;290:1566-8.

Finnerty FA Jr: Step-down treatment of mild systemic hypertension. Am J Cardiol 1984;53:1304-7.

Grimm RH, Neaton JD, McDonald M, Case J, McGill E, et al.: Beneficial effects from systematic dosage reduction of the diuretic, chlorthalidone: a randomized study within a clinical trial. Am Heart J 1985;109:858-64.

Langford HG, Blaufox MD, Oberman A, Hawkins CM, Curb JD, et al.: Dietary therapy slows the return of hypertension after stopping prolonged medication. JAMA 1985;253:657-64.

Virag R, Bouilly P, Frydman D: Is impotence an arterial disorder? Lancet 1985;1:181-4.

TABLE 7
SIDE EFFECTS OF ANTIHYPERTENSIVE DRUGS

Drugs	Side Effects	Precautions and Special Considerations
Thiazides and related	Hypokalemia, hyperuricemia, glucose intolerance, hypercholesterolemia, hypertriglyceridemia	May be ineffective in renal failure; hypokalemia increases digitalis toxicity; and hyperuricemia may precipitate acute gout
Loop diuretics	Same as for thiazides	Effective in chronic renal failure; hyponatremia, especially in the elderly
Potassium-sparing agents	Hyperkalemia	Danger of hyperkalemia in patients with renal failure
Amiloride		
Spironolactone	Gynecomastia, mastodynia	
Triamterene		

Peripheral-acting adrenergic inhibitors		
Guanadrel	Orthostatic hypotension and diarrhea	Use cautiously in elderly patients because of orthostatic hypotension
Guanethidine	Same as for guanadrel	Same as for guanadrel
Rauwolfia alkaloids, reserpine	Lethargy, nasal congestion	Contraindicated with history of mental depression; use with caution with history of peptic ulcer
Central-acting adrenergic inhibitors		
Clonidine	Drowsiness, dry mouth, fatigue	Rebound hypertension may occur after abrupt discontinuance
Guanabenz		Same as for clonidine
Methyldopa		May cause liver damage, positive direct Coombs' test, other auto-immune disorders
α_1-Adrenergic blocker		
Prazosin	Orthostatic hypotension, weakness, and palpitations	Delete diuretics to minimize orthostatic hypotension

(continued) ⇩

TABLE 7
SIDE EFFECTS OF ANTIHYPERTENSIVE DRUGS *(Continued)*

Drugs	Side Effects	Precautions and Special Considerations
β-Adrenergic blockers (Less in those with ISA)	Bradycardia, fatigue, insomnia, bizarre dreams, hypertriglyceridemia, decreased HDL cholesterol; exacerbation of angina, depression	Should not be used in patients with asthma, chronic obstructive pulmonary disease, congestive failure, heart block (greater than first degree), and sick sinus syndrome; use with caution in patients with diabetes and peripheral vascular disease
Combined α- and β-adrenergic blockers		
Labetalol	Asthma, nausea, fatigue, dizziness, and headache	Contraindicated in cardiac failure, chronic obstructive pulmonary disease, sick sinus syndrome, and heart block (greater than first degree); use with caution in patients with diabetes
Vasodilators	Headache, tachycardia, and fluid retention	May precipitate angina in patients with coronary heart disease
Hydralazine	Positive antinuclear antibody	Lupus syndrome may occur

Minoxidil	Hypertrichosis, fluid retention	May cause or aggravate pleural and pericardial effusions
Angiotensin-converting enzyme inhibitors	Rash and loss of taste	Can cause reversible, acute renal failure in patients with bilateral renal arterial stenosis; neutropenia may occur in patients with autoimmune-collagen disorders; and proteinuria
Slow channel calcium-entry blocking agents*	Headache, flushing, and dizziness	
Diltiazem	Nausea	Use with caution in patients with congestive failure or heart block
Nifedipine	Flushing, local edema	
Verapamil	Flushing, edema, and constipation	Same as for diltiazem

*These drugs have not yet been approved by the FDA for the treatment of hypertension.

#29 Resistant Hypertension

Volume Overload

Some patients may not respond to appropriate antihypertensive therapy because of reactive fluid retention (see Section 27). Of the multiple reasons for resistance to therapy shown in Table 8, volume overload due either to inadequate diuretic therapy or to excessive sodium intake is the most common. The problem may not become obvious until the blood pressure is partially lowered. This creates an even greater tendency for sodium retention by the hypertensive patient's kidneys, which have been re-set to tolerate a higher head of pressure without excreting extra volume. When the pressure is lowered, even to levels well within the normal range, the hypertensive patient's kidneys may respond by retaining more sodium and water in a misguided attempt to bring the pressure back to the higher level to which they have adjusted.

Therefore, blood pressures that have been successfully lowered may begin to gradually increase — a process called "pseudo tolerance" since it is caused by reactive fluid retention and not by a true tolerance or tachyphylaxis to the antihypertensive therapy. Doses of diuretic that were adequate may need to be increased. Amounts of dietary sodium that did not appear to be excessive may need to be reduced.

The problem is most common with those antihypertensive agents that stimulate the renin-aldosterone mechanism, such as direct acting vasodilators (hydralazine or minoxidil) and less common with those that suppress it, such as beta-blockers and CEIs. Calcium antagonists may actually be natriuretic and therefore less likely to cause fluid retention.

Inadequate Drugs

In addition to the need for supplementary or more potent diuretics, the doses of other antihypertensives may need to be increased either because inadequate amounts have been prescribed or because their effects are being antagonized. The doses may be too low because some patients inactivate the drugs more rapidly. The acetylation of hydralazine is genetically determined to be slow or rapid; hepatic blood flow and metabolism may be increased by other drugs, food or nicotine.

Antagonism From Other Drugs

A number of other drugs may antagonize the effects of antihypertensive agents. Some of them do so by stimulating the sympathetic nervous system, e.g. phenylpropanolamine in diet pills and nasal decongestants, amphetamine, and cocaine. Others, such as antidepressants, block the action of drugs that work via neuronal uptake, e.g. guanethidine, methyldopa. Non-steroidal anti-inflammatory drugs decrease the effects of diuretics and beta-blockers, perhaps by decreasing levels of vasodilatory prostaglandins. NSAIDs may be found to interfere with the action of captopril since this CEI has been shown to work in part by stimulating prostaglandin synthesis.

Associated Conditions

Other conditions that may elevate the blood pressure may either have been present all along and missed or have developed after therapy was begun. The importance of the pressor effect of alcohol intake greater than 2 ounces a day is described in Section 9. Renal damage from progressive nephrosclerosis is particularly common in blacks, whereas diabetics are susceptible to progressive glomerular sclerosis. As renal function deteriorates, hypertension often worsens, likely from sodium retention.

Renovascular Hypertension

Of all the secondary forms of hypertension, renovascular disease is the most common among those with resistant hypertension. As noted in Section 5, it is particularly common among those with rapidly progressive disease and was found in one-third of a series of 123 patients with accelerated or malignant hypertension.

Overview

The cause for resistant hypertension should be recognizable. It may take hospitalization but that step should only rarely be necessary and, in fact, may be misleading. The blood pressure almost always falls in the hospital but may rise again after discharge, even without obvious changes in therapy.

If the cause can be identified, relief may be simple. If not, larger doses of more potent drugs may be required.

References:

Gifford RW, Tarazi RC: Resistant hypertension: diagnosis and management. Ann Intern Med 1978;88:661-5.

Ramsay LE, Silas JH, Freestone S: Diuretic treatment of resistant hypertension. Br Med J 1980;281:1101-3.

Swales JD, Bing RF, Heagerty A, Pohl JEF, Russell GI, Thurston H: Treatment of refractory hypertension. Lancet 1982;1:894-6.

Webster J: Interactions of NSAIDs with diuretics and β-blockers: mechanisms and clinical implications. Drugs 1985;30:32-41.

TABLE 8

CAUSES OF RESISTANT HYPERTENSION

Inadequate drugs

- Doses too low
- Inappropriate combinations, e.g. two centrally-acting adrenergic inhibitors
- Rapid inactivation, e.g. hydralazine
- Incomplete absorption related to food intake
- Antagonism from other drugs
  - Sympathomimetics
  - Antidepressants
  - Adrenal steroids
  - Non-steroidal anti-inflammatory drugs

Associated conditions

- Alcohol intake above 2 oz/day
- Renal insufficiency
- Renovascular hypertension
- Pheochromocytoma

Volume overload

- Inadequate diuretic
- Excessive sodium intake
- Fluid retention from reduction of blood pressure
- Progressive renal damage

Volume depletion ⇒ increased renin ⇒ vasoconstriction

- Renal salt-wasting
- Overly aggressive diuretic therapy

#30 Special Patients: Young and Old

HYPERTENSION IN CHILDREN

Hypertension in pre-pubertal children is rare, often symptomatic and usually secondary. Hypertension in post-pubertal children and adolescents is more common, usually asymptomatic and more likely primary (or idiopathic). Since blood pressures have been taken more frequently among young people, the presence of hypertension in as many as 1% of seemingly healthy adolescents has been recognized. Different criteria for hypertension in children of various ages have been proposed in the JNC III report. These are the suggested upper limits of normal BP in children by age, from JNC III:

Age/Years	Blood Pressure
14-18	<135/90
10-14	<125/85
6-10	<120/80
<6	<110/75

Pre-Pubertal

The younger the patient with elevated blood pressure, the more likely it represents a congenital problem. These include:

- Coarctation of the aorta
- Hypoplasia of the kidney
- Congenital adrenal hyperplasia

Most advise a study of renal function and structure for every pre-pubertal child with hypertension without an obvious cause; in the past, usually an IVP, or currently ultrasound, CT or digital subtraction arteriography.

Post-Pubertal

The older the child, the more likely hypertension is primary. Obesity is a major factor and weight reduction should be the first approach to therapy. Guidelines as to when to institute drug therapy and which drug should be used remain unsettled. Some believe that evidence of left ventricular hypertrophy by echocardiography, present in a surprisingly high percentage of adolescents with presumably mild hypertension, is an indication for the use of drug therapy. More information is needed since some LVH may be a necessary response to the elevated afterload from increased vascular resistance.

HYPERTENSION IN THE ELDERLY

As many as half of people over 65 will develop systolic hypertension, defined as a BP above 160 mm Hg. People who develop significant diastolic hypertension after age 60 should be evaluated for renovascular disease. Isolated systolic hypertension reflects increasing atherosclerotic rigidity of large arteries. Some who have very high cuff blood pressure readings may have "pseudohypertension" from inability of the balloon to compress the calcified brachial artery. Such falsely high readings should be suspected if the radial artery remains palpable after the Korotkoff sounds disappear (Osler's sign).

The presence of isolated systolic levels above 160 mm Hg is associated with an increased risk of stroke and other cardiovascular disease. However, little data are available as to the ability of antihypertensive therapy to lower such pressures or to remove the risks of CVD. A placebo-controlled study, Systolic Hypertension in the Elderly Program, has just been started.

Therapy

Elderly people with diastolic levels above 95 mm Hg should be treated since they are protected as well, if not better, than younger patients by appropriate therapy. Non-drugs, as described in Sections 9 and 10,should be tried since elderly people may have more problems with drugs due to various age-related changes, including the following:

- Loss of baroreceptor responsiveness, increasing their propensity to postural hypotension
- Decrease in myocardial contractility
- Shrinkage of body fluid volume
- Decrease in renal excretory capacity
- Inability to remember doses and to open child-resistant bottles of drugs

They are more likely to have other medical problems which may be aggravated by antihypertensive therapy, e.g. diabetes by diuretics or β-blockers, or which involve the use of medications which may interfere with the therapy of hypertension, e.g. NSAIDs with the action of diuretic or β-blockers.

The types of drugs used in the elderly need to be carefully considered. Doses of diuretics should be minimized so as not to decrease further a shrunken fluid volume but should be adequate to overcome reduced renal capacity to excrete sodium. Central agonists may further reduce mental alertness; beta-blockers may interfere with sleep and physical alertness. Initial exeriences with calcium antagonists have shown them to be particularly effective in the elderly.

Drugs should be given cautiously, with the initial goal of gradually and gently lowering systolic BP to below 160 mm Hg and diastolic BP to below 95 mm Hg.

References:

Finnegan TP, Spence JD, Wong DG, Wells GA: Blood pressure measurement in the elderly: correlation of arterial stiffness with difference between intra-arterial and cuff pressures. J Hypertension 1985;3:231-5.

Hofman A, Valkenburgh HA, Maas J, Groustra FN: The natural history of blood pressure in childhood. Int J Epidemiol 1985;14:91-6.

Hulley SB, Furberg CD, Gurland B, et al.: Systolic hypertension in the Elderly Program (SHEP): antihypertensive efficacy of chlorthalidone. Am J Cardiol 1985;56:913-20.

Lipsitz LA, Storch HA, Minaker KL, Rowe JW: Intraindividual variability in postural blood pressure in the elderly. Clin Sci 1985;69:337-41.

Messerli FH, Ventura HO, Amodeo C: Osler's maneuver and pseudohypertension. N Engl J Med 1985;312:1548-51.

#31 Special Patients: Diabetics

Hypertension is more common among patients with diabetes and poses a major threat to the kidneys. The treatment of hypertension may aggravate glucose tolerance and interfere with the recovery from insulin-induced hypoglycemia. Obviously diabetic hypertensives are a large and difficult group to manage.

The Association Between Diabetes and Hypertension

Hypertension is more common among diabetics, in some studies twice more common than among non-diabetics. The following increase the likelihood of hypertension:

- Older age
- Longer duration of diabetes
- Presence of proteinuria
- Obesity
- Female gender

Not only is hypertension more common among overt diabetics but it is also more common among those with normal fasting blood sugars but abnormal glucose tolerance tests. Such patients tend to be more obese. Obesity, hypertension and glucose intolerance may all reflect tissue insulin resistance.

Various diabetic complications may be accelerated by hypertension. The most striking acceleration has been in the progression of diabetic glomerulosclerosis or Kimmelstiel-Wilson disease which has become a major cause for end-stage renal disease (ESRD) as diabetics survive longer. Experimental data show that glomerular sclerosis is accelerated by hyperperfusion of the capillary bed, as would be induced by high osmotic pressure from hyperglycemia and high intravascular pressure from hypertension. As will be noted, the progression of renal insufficiency has been slowed by effective antihypertensive therapy.

Therapy of Hypertension in Diabetics

The blood pressure should be carefully controlled to prevent the progression of diabetic renal disease. Successful control of hypertension has been shown to slow the progressive fall in glomerular filtration rate and the amount of albuminuria in diabetics with nephropathy.

Problems With Drugs

Unfortunately, diabetics may be susceptible to various additional problems with many of the currently available antihypertensives. These include:

- Diuretics, which may worsen glucose tolerance and raise fasting blood sugars, probably by inducing hypokalemia which may decrease insulin secretion and/or effect
- Beta-blockers, which may blunt the effects of epinephrine needed to overcome insulin-induced hypoglycemia
- Both diuretics and beta-blockers may cause further derangements in blood lipids which are often abnormal in diabetics

- Drugs such as central agonists and alpha-blockers may cause more postural hypotension
- CEIs may lead to more glomerular damage since they may cause a glomerulopathy, although this effect has not been shown to occur more frequently in diabetics given CEIs. CEIs have been found to reduce proteinuria and renal damage better than other anti-hypertensive drugs in hypertensive animals
- No hyperglycemic effect has been noted from the use of calcium antagonists although they may interfere with the release of insulin

Therapy Guidelines

Non-insulin dependent diabetics may be safely treated with any antihypertensive agent but should be monitored for worsening of hyperglycemia and hyperlipidemia. Diuretic-induced hypokalemia should be prevented if possible and corrected if it occurs.

Insulin dependent diabetics should not be given beta-blockers.

All diabetics should be carefully checked for microalbuminuria. If it is present, patients should be carefully controlled with the hope of preventing the progression of glomerulosclerosis.

References:

Cederholm J, Wibell L: Glucose intolerance in middle-aged subjects - a cause of hypertension? Acta Med Scand 1985;217:363-71.

Klein R, Klein BE, Moss SE, DeMets DL: Blood pressure and hypertension in diabetes. Am J Epidemiol 1985;122:75-89.

Krolewski AS, Warram JH, Cupples A, Gorman CK, Szabo AJ, Christlieb AR: Hypertension, orthostatic hypotension and the microvascular complications of diabetes. J Chron Dis 1985;38:319-26.

Parving H-H, Andersen AR, Smidt UM, Svendsen PAA: Early aggressive antihypertensive treatment reduces rate of decline in kidney function in diabetic nephropathy. Lancet 1983;1:1175-9.

Taguma Y, Kitamoto Y, Futaki G, et al.: Effect of captopril on heavy proteinuria in azotemic diabetics. N Engl J Med 1985;313:1617-20.

#32 Special Patients: Coronary or Cerebral Vascular Disease

Hypertension is the major risk factor for both coronary and cerebral vascular disease. Antihypertensive therapy will reduce the incidence of mortality from stroke. Protection from coronary disease by previously used therapies has not been conclusively demonstrated (see Section 11).

This section will examine the management of hypertension in patients with either coronary or cerebral vascular disease.

CORONARY ARTERY DISEASE AND HYPERTENSION

Hypertensive patients with chronic stable angina should not be given direct vasodilators (hydralazine or minoxidil) unless the propensity of these drugs to stimulate sympathetic reflexes is covered by concomitant therapy with adrenergic inhibitors.

Hypertensive patients with atypical angina due to coronary spasm given beta-blockers may be susceptible to unopposed alpha-mediated vasoconstriction, although their reduction in myocardial work usually leads to reduction in anginal attacks.

Patients early in the course of an acute myocardial infarction may have a marked hypertensive response from pain and stress-induced surges in catecholamine discharge. If the pressure remains very high despite relief of pain and anxiety, careful reduction of BP may be attempted under careful monitoring. Early use of beta-blockers has been advocated to reduce the extent of myocardial damage and may be used to also lower the BP. Unfortunately, the immediate antihypertensive effect of beta-blockers is usually minimal. Intravenous nitroglycerin or a calcium antagonist may be better choices.

After the early period, continued use of oral beta-blockers has been shown to reduce recurrent MIs and mortality. Some patients who were hypertensive before an MI have a marked fall in BP post-MI, which may be a bad prognostic sign if it reflects impaired myocardial function.

REVERSAL OF LVH

In addition to the use of beta-blockers and calcium antagonists to reduce myocardial work and improve coronary blood flow in patients with coronary disease, various antihypertensive drugs have been shown to reverse the left ventricular hypertrophy that is frequently noted by echocardiography, even in patients with relatively mild hypertension. Reversal has been seen with virtually all adrenergic inhibitors but not so uniformly with either diuretics or direct vasodilators.

CONGESTIVE HEART FAILURE

Various vasodilators have been found to reduce afterload and improve myocardial function in patients with CHF. The most impressive and sustained improvement has been noted with CEIs and CHF is a major indication for the use of captopril.

CEREBRAL VASCULAR DISEASE

Antihypertensive therapy has uniformly been found to reduce mortality from strokes. Despite occassional reports of overly aggressive therapy producing either transient or permanent ischemic brain damage, the proper use of antihypertensive therapy is clearly indicated in patients with hypertension in association with TIAs or after a CVA.

ACUTE STROKE

Caution is needed in the management of patients during the early course of a stroke. They may have transient rises in BP, presumably reflecting irritation of vasomotor centers or non-specific responses to stress. Such rises may need to be gently lowered under careful monitoring, preferably with nitroprusside, particularly if the patient is having intracranial hemorrhage. However, if the blood pressure is lowered and brain function deteriorates, the pressure should be allowed to rise to ensure that blood flow is not being further reduced.

CHRONIC THERAPY

Cerebral blood flow (CBF) is kept very stable by adrenergically-regulated changes in the caliber of cerebral arteries and arterioles. The range of cerebral autoregulation in normotensive people is roughly between 70/40 and 180/110 mm Hg. Levels below the lower limits induce a fall in CBF with signs and symptoms of "shock"; levels above the upper limits induce hyperperfusion of the brain that is responsible for hypertensive encephalopathy (see Section 34).

Patients with chronic hypertension have a shift to the right of the entire curve, reflecting the structural thickening of cerebral arteries. The range wherein autoregulation maintains normal CBF may then be between 140/90 and 210/130. Sudden lowering of BP to below 140/90, though certainly not to a truly hypotensive level, may nonetheless induce cerebral hypoperfusion and bring on postural dizziness, weakness and faintness.

Fortunately, the range of cerebral autoregulation shifts back to the left with time, after persistent and gradual lowering of BP, presumably reflecting a decrease in the thickness of cerebral arteries. Thereby, lower levels of BP, well into the truly normotensive range, may then be tolerated. These findings may explain the frequent "washed-out" feeling that patients have when first using too much antihypertensive therapy that works too well. The better course is to go slow, bringing BP down only 5 to 10 mm Hg at a time, hopefully allowing CBF to be well maintained.

References:

Barry DI: Cerebral blood flow in hypertension. J Cardiovasc Pharmacol 1985;7:S94-8.

Bayliss J, Norell MS, Canepa-Anson R, Reid C, Poole-Wilson P, Sutton G: Clinical importance of the renin-angiotensin system in chronic heart failure: double blind comparison of captopril and prazosin. Br Med J 1985;290:1861-6.

Schlant RC: Reversal of left ventricular hypertrophy by drug treatment of hypertension. Chest 1985;88 (Suppl):194S-8S.

Strandgaard S, Paulson OB: Cerebral autoregulation. Stroke 1984;15:413-6.

Wallace JD, Levy LL: Blood pressure after stroke. JAMA 1981;246:2177-80.

#33 Special Patients: Renal Insufficency

As noted in Section 5, progressive renal insufficiency is a common consequence of sustained hypertension, particularly in blacks who often have more nephrosclerosis than whites with similar degrees of hypertension. Half of blacks who reach end-stage renal disease (ESRD) that requires dialysis therapy do so as a result of hypertension. Although a smaller proportion of whites develop ESRD from their hypertension, this remains the most common preventable type of ESRD.

The development of renal insufficiency tends to aggravate hypertension and may cause it de novo. Approximately 85% of patients with renal insufficiency will have hypertension, setting up the cycle: renal damage causes hypertension which causes renal damage. The process may involve sodium retention in most and the hypersecretion of renin in some. Patients with interstitial nephritis have less hypertension, probably because they waste sodium. Patients with collagen vascular diseases may have rapidly accelerating hypertension because the intra-renal vascular disease activates renin release.

THE TREATMENT OF HYPERTENSION

Control of Fluid Volume

Control of sodium intake and excretion become increasingly more important as renal function worsens. Dietary sodium restriction should help, with the caution that overly rigorous restriction may cause those who have a fixed degree of sodium wastage to become volume depleted. Diuretics are almost always needed. Thiazides generally work only if the GFR is above 30 ml/min, reflected in a serum creatinine below 2.5 mg/dl. Those with more severe renal insufficiency will usually require a loop diuretic, although metolazone will work in many and requires only once a day dosage (see Section 14).

Other Therapy

In addition to adequate diuretic therapy, a number of other antihypertensive drugs may be tried, with no clear superiority of any other except for minoxidil. Most reserve this drug for those with severe hypertension, but it may prove useful in milder disease as well. CEIs may also be useful, particularly among those with a renin component to their hypertension. As noted in Section 23, renal function may suddenly worsen in patients given CEIs if previous high levels of angiotensin II were maintaining renal perfusion. This is most likely to occur in patients with bilateral renovascular disease or with a stenosis in the artery to a solitary kidney.

Overly aggressive falls in BP from any drug may at least transiently reduce renal blood flow and cause the serum creatinine to rise further. If the rise is not progressive or excessive, therapy should be continued since successful long-term control of hypertension may lead to an improvement of renal function. Such improvement has been noted less commonly than hoped for, perhaps because drugs have been used which further constrict renal vessels. Hopefully the use of vasodilators such as CEIs or calcium blockers will provide better protection of renal function.

Doses of Drugs

Most antihypertensive drugs can be given in usual doses to patients with renal insufficiency. Exceptions include methyldopa, clonidine, the water-soluble beta-blockers (atenolol and nadolol), and captopril whose doses should be reduced by half or more in the presence of renal insufficiency.

Dialysis and Transplantation

When renal function nears the end, dialysis is usually necessary to bring the blood pressure under control. In some, the response is dramatic. Hypertension that was unmanageable on 3 or 4 medications may become easily controlled on small doses of 1 or 2. In others, however, the blood pressure remains a problem, particularly on the days between dialyses. More careful dialysis by the chronic peritoneal route may provide better control of hypertension.

Post Transplant

The implantation of a normal kidney may relieve or cure hypertension even if it began as the primary (idiopathic) form. This suggests that primary hypertension may start from renal dysfunction. Unfortunately, a number of events in the post-transplant period may bring hypertension back. These include cyclosporin therapy, high doses of steroids, rejection and stenoses at the graft site.

References:

Anderson S, Meyer TW, Rennke HG, Brenner BM: Control of glomerular hypertension limits glomerular injury in rats with reduced renal mass. J Clin Invest 1985;76:612-19.

Bennett WM, Muther RS, Parker RA, et al.: Drug therapy in renal failure: dosing guidelines for adults. Ann Intern Med 1980;93:286-325.

Curtis JJ, Luke RG, Jones P, Diethelm AG, Whelchel JD: Hypertension after successful renal transplantation. Am J Med 1985;79:193-200.

Mourad G, Mimran A, Mion CM: Recovery of renal function in patients with accelerated malignant nephrosclerosis on maintenance dialysis with management of blood pressure by captopril. Nephron 1985;41:166-9.

Wollam GL, Tarazi RC, Bravo EL, Dustan HP: Diuretic potency of combined hydrochlorothiazide and furosemide therapy in patients with azotemia. Am J Med 1982;72:929-37.

#34 Treatment of Hypertensive Crises

Some patients with markedly elevated blood pressures may pose a therapeutic emergency. Their blood pressure may need to be reduced within minutes, if there is immediate danger to brain, heart or large vessel integrity; or within hours, if blood pressure is so high as to pose an eventual threat to vascular and target organ function. It is useful to segregate hypertensive "emergencies" from "urgencies" in selecting the best therapy:

- Hypertensive emergencies:
  - Hypertensive encephalopathy, including eclampsia
  - Severe hypertension in the presence of active myocardial ischemia
  - Intracranial hemorrhage or dissecting aneurysms
  - Hypertension in the immediate post-operative period
- Hypertensive urgencies:
  - Accelerated (Grade 3 fundi) or malignant (Grade 4) hypertension
  - Diastolic levels above 140 mm Hg
  - Congestive heart failure
  - Cerebral thrombosis
  - Rapidly advancing renal ischemia, e.g. scleroderma crisis
  - Intractable nose bleed
  - MAO-tyramine interaction
  - Sympathomimetic drug overdose
  - Rebound from abrupt cessation of adrenergic inhibiting drugs

Drugs For Hypertensive Emergencies

When feasible, such patients should be admitted to an intensive care unit, have an intra-arterial line inserted for constant monitoring of BP, and started on an I.V. drip of nitroprusside. They should have the diastolic BP lowered to a safe level, usually below 120 mm Hg, to remove the immediate danger but not so low as to reduce blood flow to vital organs. The safe diastolic level likely will be above 100 mm Hg. If evidence of brain or heart ischemia develop, the pressure can quickly be allowed to rise to see if the lower pressure is responsible. If not, the diastolic pressure should be kept between 100 and 120 mm Hg. Appropriate anti-hypertensive drugs should be started for more chronic therapy if the patient can take oral medication. I.V. furosemide may be needed to overcome the tendency toward fluid retention with successful lowering of the blood pressure. However, diuretics may not be indicated initially, and may actually be contraindicated, if the patient's fluid volume is depleted from prior GI or renal losses.

If nitroprusside is not indicated or feasible, I.V. labetalol or diazoxide given by slow continuous infusion or repeated mini-bolus injections will usually provide fast and adequate reduction of the blood pressure. Caution is needed not to reduce pressure too fast or too much.

Drugs For Hypertensive Urgencies

Patients in less tenuous condition but with markedly high pressures have been successfully treated with numerous oral agents including clonidine, prazosin, captopril and even minoxidil. Nifedipine, either placed under the tongue or swallowed, has been found to be particularly effective in rapidly bringing very high pressures down quickly and smoothly. Only 10 mg is usually needed but that dose may be repeated in 30 minutes if an inadequate response to the initial dose is noted. Some will experience too precipitous a fall with the initial dose and a more slowly absorbed form of the drug as is available in Europe might be even safer. Captopril may also be used sublingually.

The goal of therapy is not simply to lower the high pressures but to institute an effective regimen for long-term control that the patient will take. This may require two or three oral drugs, as covered in Sections 26 and 27. They can be started in small doses as soon as the pressure has been brought down from dangerously high levels and the patient returned within 1 or 2 days to ensure that control is being achieved. As with all hypertensive patients, particularly with those who have lesser elevations, these patients should have the pressure brought down in a steady and gradual manner so as not to reduce cerebral and other organ blood flows too much, thereby making the patient dizzy, weak and sedated.

Evaluation For Causes

Patients seen for hypertensive crisis must have a careful examination to uncover the underlying cause. Some may be obvious; however, renovascular disease is responsible in a significant number of patients and a renal arteriogram should be done in all who do not have another obvious cause.

References:

Ahmed MEK, Walker JM, Beevers DG, Beevers M: Lack of difference between malignant and accelerated hypertension. Br Med J 1986;292:235-7.

Bertel O, Conen D, Radü EW, Müller J, Lang C, Dubach UC: Nifedipine in hypertensive emergencies. Br Med J 1983;286:19-21.

Ferguson RK, Vlasses PH: Hypertensive emergencies and urgencies. JAMA 1986;255:1607-13.

Hauger-Klevene JH: Comparison of sublingual captopril and nifedipine. Lancet 1986;1:219.

Jarden JO, Barry DI, Juhler M, Graham DI, Strandgaard S, Paulson OB: Cerebrovascular aspects of converting-enzyme inhibition II: blood-brain barrier permeability and effect of intracerebroventricular administration of captopril. J. Hypertension 1984;2:599-604.

Lebel M, Langlois S, Belleau LJ, Grose JH: Labetalol infusion in hypertensive emergencies. Clin Pharmacol Ther 1985;37:615-8.

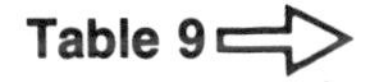

TABLE 9
DRUGS FOR HYPERTENSIVE CRISES

Drug	Dosage	Onset of Action	Adverse Effects
Vasodilators			
Nitroprusside (Nipride, Nitropress)	0.5-10 microgram/kg/min as IV infusion	Instantaneous	Nausea, vomiting, muscle twitching, sweating, thiocyanate intoxication
Nitroglycerin	5-100 microgram/min as IV infusion	2-5 min	Bradycardia, tachycardia, flushing, headache, vomiting, methemoglobinemia
Diazoxide (Hyperstat)	50-100 mg as IV bolus, repeated or 15-30 mg/min by IV infusion	2-4 min	Nausea, hypotension, flushing, tachycardia, chest pain
Hydralazine (Apresoline)	10-20 mg IV 10-50 mg IM	10 min 20-30 min	Tachycardia, flushing, headache, vomiting, aggravation of angina

Adrenergic inhibitors			
Phentolamine (Regitine)	5-15 mg IV	1-2 min	Tachycardia, flushing
Trimethaphan (Arfonad)	1-4 mg/min as IV infusion	5-10 min	Paresis of bowel and bladder, orthostatic hypotension, blurred vision, dry mouth
Labetalol (Normodyne, Trandate)	20-80 mg IV bolus every 10 minutes 2 mg/min IV infusion	5-10 min	Vomiting, scalp tingling, burning in throat and groin, postural hypotension, dizziness, nausea
Methyldopa (Aldomet)	250-500 mg IV infusion	2-3 hours	Drowsiness